How to prepare
for MRCOG
Part 2

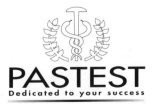

PASTEST
Dedicated to your success

Editor's details:

Austin Ugwumadu MBBS MRCOG
Consultant Obstetrician & Gynaecologist
& Honorary Senior Lecturer
St George's Hospital
London

Authors' details:

Charlotte Chaliha MA MD MRCOG
Subspeciality trainee in Urogynaecology
St Mary's Hospital
London

Barry Whitlow MD MRCOG
Consultant Obstetrician & Gynaecologist
Essex Rivers Trust
Colchester Hospital
Turner Road
Colchester
Essex

Andrea Hermann MD DFFP MRCOG MRCPI
Consultant Gynaecologist
Galway Clinic
Doughiska
Co. Galway
Ireland

How to prepare for MRCOG
Part 2

Charlotte Chaliha

Barry Whitlow

Andrea Hermann

Edited by Austin Ugwumadu

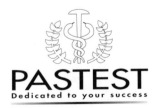

PASTEST
Dedicated to your success

© 2004 PasTest
Egerton Court
Parkgate Estate
Knutsford
Cheshire WAI6 8DX

Telephone: 01565 752000

First edition 2004

ISBN: 1 901198 51 0

A catalogue record for this book is available from the British Library.

Text prepared by Saxon Graphics Ltd, Derby
Printed and bound in Great Britain by Page Bros (Norwich Ltd).
Cover design by OldTinDog.com

Contents

Introduction

The Part 2 examination is designed to test the candidate's theoretical and practical knowledge of obstetrics and gynaecology as well as his/her knowledge of the scientific foundations of the specialty. Possession of this knowledge is essential but not enough to pass unless the candidate can demonstrate that he or she can and has indeed applied this knowledge to the management of clinical problems. In recent years, the format for testing candidates has undergone significant changes and now demands concise and evidence based answers to controversial questions. Essentially, the Royal College wants to know your opinion/approach (as a prospective member) to these controversial questions.

The aim of this book is to assist candidates preparing for the Part 2 MRCOG examination. It features:

- 2 Multiple Choice Question practice papers with explanations

- 25 short essay questions divided between obstetrics and gynaecology; and

- 24 OSCE stations equivalent to two practice exams.

The sample questions and answers cover the range of subject material and clinical scenarios commonly encountered in the Part 2 exam. They are set at the minimum standard expected of the membership candidate and the authors recommend that readers attempt the questions before consulting the model answers.

Austin Ugwumadu, Consultant/Hon Senior Lecturer in Obstetrics & Gynaecology

The structure of the Part 2 MRCOG examination

1. Written paper consisting of:

- 300 MCQ questions; and
- 2 short essay papers divided into

    Paper 1 – five obstetric questions and

    Paper 2 – five gynaecology questions

2. Objective Structured Clinical Examination (OSCE), which consists of 12 stations lasting 15 minutes each.

Syllabus for Part 2 MRCOG

The syllabus for Part 2 examination as published by the Royal College of Obstetricians and Gynaecologists is now summarised.

Genetics and Embryology

Comprehensive knowledge of normal and abnormal karyotypes, the inheritance of genetic disorders, the genetic causes of infertility and early abortion, as well as the ability to transmit this knowledge to patients, to discuss its implications as well as any ethical dilemmas.

Anatomy

Continuing comprehensive knowledge of anatomy, particularly as applied to surgical procedures undertaken by the obstetrician and gynaecologist.

Pathology, Biochemistry and Endocrinology

Thorough knowledge of the pathology of the genital tract and associated structures; sound understanding of biochemistry of mother and fetus, together with indepth knowledge of metabolism. While endocrinological knowledge of all organs is required extensive knowledge is expected of the endocrine organs as applied to reproductive medicine.

Pharmacology

Comprehensive knowledge of all aspects of pharmacology is required with particular knowledge of those drugs which will be used in obstetrics and gynaecology.

Immunology

Candidates are expected to understand basic immunology and how this may be changed in pregnancy; fetal development of the immune system, with particular knowledge of rhesus and other isoimmunisations.

Infectious diseases

Comprehensive knowledge of the infectious diseases affecting pregnant and non-pregnant females as well as the fetus *in utero*. Knowledge of epidemiology, diagnostic techniques, prophylaxis, immunisation and the use of antibiotics and antiviral agents.

Epidemiology and Statistics

Candidates should understand how to apply statistical analysis, to collect data; have knowledge of setting up of clinical trials and the ability to interpret data.

Normal pregnancy

Knowledge of all maternal and fetal systems. Comprehensive knowledge of antepartum care, its aims and method of implementation. Similarly, with intrapartum care, which should include in-depth knowledge of obstetric analgesia and anaesthesia.

Abnormal pregnancy

Clear knowledge of all aspects of abnormality both in pregnancy, labour and puerperium is expected together with their management. Detailed knowledge of neonatal resuscitation is mandatory.

Pre- and post-pregnancy counselling

Candidates should demonstrate their ability to advise patients regarding any aspect of obstetric or gynaecological disease.

Maternal and perinatal mortality

Candidates are expected to be familiar with the definitions and concepts as well as to be conversant with confidential enquiries into maternal deaths and the reports on birth surveys.

Gynaecology

Proficiency in history taking in general and gynaecology in particular, and at general and gynaecological examination. Detailed knowledge of all basic gynaecological procedures as well as the ability to perform more common gynaecological operations is required. Candidates will be expected to have a knowledge of more complicated procedures, eg in oncology, though at the level of the Membership examination proficiency in these areas will not be expected.

Prepubertal gynaecology

Thorough knowledge of normal and abnormal sexual development, paediatric pathology and its management, normal puberty, and its disorders.

Disorders of menstruation

Based on the physiology of normal menstruation, in-depth understanding of pathophysiology of menstrual disorders, their investigation and management. The menopause.

Infertility

Causes, investigation and management of infertility together with basic knowledge in the techniques involved in *in vitro* fertilisation.

Contraception and Abortion

All methods of contraception should be thoroughly understood and candidates are obliged to present evidence of practical experience. The reasons for, techniques and complications of performing therapeutic abortion should be understood.

Psychosexual Medicine

A thorough understanding of the principles of psychosexual medicine is required.

Gynaecological Oncology

The epidemiology and aetiology of gynaecological tumours. The principles of carcinogenesis, tumour immunology and pathology together with diagnostic techniques and staging of gynaecological tumours is essential. Basic principles of treatment, both surgery, radiotherapy and chemotherapy together with knowledge of terminal care from gynaecological malignancy.

Multiple-choice questions (MCQs)

Paper 1

Gynaecology

Indicate your answers with a T (True) or F (False) in the box provided. The answers for this section start on page 227.

Regarding cervical screening

1 The screening programme targets women between 20 and 50 years of age.
2 Pap smear tests have a false-negative rate of 15–25%.
3 The incidence of mild dyskaryosis is approximately 10%.
4 The incidence of moderate dyskaryosis is 5%.
5 The incidence of severe dyskaryosis is 0.5%.

Risk factors for anal sphincter injury are

6 Midline episiotomy.
7 Prolonged second stage of labour.
8 Fetal macrosomia.
9 Occipitoposterior position.
10 Elective Caesarean section.

Faecal incontinence

11 Is commoner in women than men.
12 Occurs in 1% of women after vaginal delivery.
13 Increases with age.
14 Pudendal neuropathy after childbirth is the most significant aetiological factor.

In a woman with a history of a previous third-degree tear, the risk of faecal incontinence after another vaginal delivery

☐ 15 Is reduced by elective episiotomy.

☐ 16 Is related to the degree of pudendal neuropathy.

☐ 17 Is increased if the woman is symptomatic.

☐ 18 Is reduced by perineal massage.

In a woman with a history of stress incontinence

☐ 19 Alpha-agonists have been shown to reduce the number of stress-incontinence episodes.

☐ 20 Conservative treatment achieves long-term cure in the majority.

☐ 21 Electrical stimulation acts by stimulation of the autonomic nerve supply.

☐ 22 Estrogen therapy has been shown to reduce symptoms.

Concerning the surgical management of stress incontinence

☐ 23 An anterior repair will correct incontinence as well as a coexistent cystocele.

☐ 24 The tension-free vaginal tape procedure has a similar success rate to Burch colposuspension.

☐ 25 The Marshall–Martchetti–Krantz and Burch colposuspension procedures will correct a coexistent cystocele.

☐ 26 A Burch colposuspension will worsen a coexistent rectocele or enterocele.

☐ 27 Needle suspension procedures have a long-term success rate of approximately 50–60%.

With regard to premature ovarian failure

☐ 28 The incidence is about 5%.

☐ 29 Occurs in 50% of patients presenting with secondary amenorrhoea.

☐ 30 Hot flushes occur in about 50% of patients.

☐ 31 Symptoms are related to the levels of LH and FSH.

☐ 32 Is associated with pelvic tuberculosis.

Regarding azoospermia

☐ 32 Two-thirds of cases are due to genital tract obstruction.

☐ 33 Obstructive azoospermia is seen in about 50% of men with cystic fibrosis.

☐ 34 Testicular biopsy samples show reduced spermatogenesis in obstructive spermatogenesis.

☐ 35 Karyotyping is always recommended in cases of azoospermia.

☐ 36 It is seen in 30% of infertile men.

In cases involving ovarian accidents

☐ 37 Among surgically managed cases, the frequency of malignant tumours is about 45% in premenopausal women and about 13% in postmenopausal women.

☐ 38 About 25% of cases of torsion occur in children.

☐ 39 Cystadenomas are the commonest tumours leading to torsion.

☐ 40 Around 15% of ovarian torsions involve ovarian malignancy.

In cases of haemorrhage into or from ovarian cysts

☐ 41 Rupture occurs most commonly on day 3–5 of the menstrual cycle.

☐ 42 Two-thirds of cases involve the right ovary.

☐ 43 The risk is increased by anticoagulants despite normal coagulation indices.

☐ 44 May cause haemolytic jaundice.

Factors that increase the risk of ovarian hyperstimulation syndrome include

☐ 45 Older age.

☐ 46 A higher number of mature and immature follicles.

☐ 47 Use of HCG for luteal support.

☐ 48 Pregnancy.

☐ 49 Higher body mass index.

Regarding assisted reproduction

☐ 50 Multiple pregnancy is more common with superovulation with/without intrauterine insemination than IVF/ICSI cycles.

☐ 51 There is a higher risk of infants of low birth weight.

☐ 52 The heterotopic pregnancy rate is about 5% in IVF pregnancies.

☐ 53 The ectopic pregnancy rate is about 15%.

The following statements regarding clomifene citrate are correct

☐ 54 The ovulation rate in a normally estrogenised woman is approximately 50%.

☐ 55 The pregnancy rate is 30–40%.

☐ 56 Side-effects are dose-dependent.

☐ 57 The use of clomifene citrate results in a 20% increase in endogenous FSH and LH concentrations.

Gonadotrophin-releasing hormone (GnRH) analogues

☐ 58 Are synthesised by substitution of amino acids at positions 4 and 8 of the decapeptide GnRH.

☐ 59 GnRH analogues lead to a higher rate of ovulation and conception than gonadotrophin regimes.

☐ 60 Most women will be hypoestrogenic within a week.

☐ 61 Any reduction in bone density is reversible after stopping treatment.

Biochemical changes seen in congenital adrenal hyperplasia due to 21-hydroxylase deficiency include

- ☐ 62 Increased urinary ketosteroids.
- ☐ 63 Increased serum aldosterone.
- ☐ 64 Decreased serum testosterone.
- ☐ 65 Increased serum 17-hydroxyprogesterone.

The following metabolic changes are seen after the menopause

- ☐ 66 A rise in plasma testosterone.
- ☐ 67 A rise in plasma calcium.
- ☐ 68 A decrease in plasma androstenedione.
- ☐ 69 A decrease in plasma cholesterol.

The following are seen in association with Turner's syndrome

- ☐ 70 Lymphoedema.
- ☐ 71 Hypogonadotrophic hypogonadism.
- ☐ 72 A single Barr body.
- ☐ 73 Increased incidence with maternal age.
- ☐ 74 Horseshoe kidney.

Hyperprolactinaemia

- ☐ 75 Occurs in 25% of patients with hyperthyroidism.
- ☐ 76 Occurs in 25% of patients with acromegaly.
- ☐ 77 May be associated with renal failure.
- ☐ 78 Is a side-effect of metoclopramide use.
- ☐ 79 Pituitary causes are mainly due to prolactin-secreting microadenomas.

Recurrent miscarriage

- [ ] 80 Is associated with diabetes.
- [ ] 81 Is increased in women with hyperthyroidism.
- [ ] 82 Antiphospholipid antibodies are present in about 15% of women.
- [ ] 83 Robertsonian translocations are the most frequent parental chromosomal abnormality.
- [ ] 84 Without treatment, women with antiphospholipid syndrome have an 85–90% risk of miscarriage.

Precocious puberty

- [ ] 85 Is defined as the onset of puberty before 8 years of age in girls.
- [ ] 86 May be a feature of neurofibromatosis.
- [ ] 87 May be caused by Cushing's disease.
- [ ] 88 May be caused by hyperthyroidism.
- [ ] 89 Basal gonadotrophin levels are elevated in true precocious puberty.

In women with hirsutism

- [ ] 90 Total serum testosterone levels are usually raised.
- [ ] 91 Serum testosterone levels correlate well with the severity of hirsutism.
- [ ] 92 Circulating dehydroepiandrosterone (sulphate DHAs) level is usually raised.
- [ ] 93 Polycystic ovarian syndrome is the commonest cause.
- [ ] 94 Most androgen-secreting tumours are benign.

Regarding the progesterone-only pill

- [ ] 95 50% of women will continue to ovulate.
- [ ] 96 Follicular development is inhibited in only 10–20% of women.
- [ ] 97 The half-life is approximately 8 hours.
- [ ] 98 The failure rate is higher in those with a low body mass index.
- [ ] 99 Is associated with an increase in functional ovarian cysts.

Risk factors for osteoporosis include

☐ 100 Early menopause.

☐ 101 Hypothyroidism.

☐ 102 Cigarette smoking.

☐ 103 Type-1 diabetes.

☐ 104 Hypergonadism.

The following drugs are associated with hyperprolactinaemia

☐ 105 Haloperidol.

☐ 106 Prochlorperazine.

☐ 107 Bromocriptine.

☐ 108 Methyldopa.

☐ 109 Cimetidine.

Plasma gonadotrophin levels are increased in

☐ 110 Turner's syndrome.

☐ 111 Kallmann's syndrome.

☐ 112 Testicular feminisation syndrome.

☐ 113 McCune–Albright syndrome.

☐ 114 Anorexia nervosa.

In cervical intraepithelial neoplasia

☐ 115 Over 99% of cases contain HPV.

☐ 116 HPV subtypes-12 and -14 are high-risk for CIN.

☐ 117 60% of CIN3 lesions progress to cancer within 10 years.

☐ 118 The HPV virus is a non-enveloped RNA virus.

☐ 119 Regions E3 and E4 code for oncoproteins.

Risk factors for cervical cancer and CIN include

☐ 120 Nulliparity.

☐ 121 Cigarette smoking.

☐ 122 Previous CIN.

☐ 123 Presence of other genital tract neoplasia.

☐ 124 High alcohol intake.

Cervical intraepithelial neoplasia

☐ 125 Usually affects the epithelium but not the gland crypts.

☐ 126 In CIN3 the mean depth of crypt involvement is over 5 mm.

☐ 127 Nuclear abnormalities are the most important feature in assessing severity.

In cervical adenocarcinoma *in situ*/(CGIN) cervical glandular intraepithelial neoplasia

☐ 128 There are no specific colposcopic features.

☐ 129 75% of patients show a glandular abnormality on cytology.

☐ 130 In one-third of cases there is an invasive squamous lesion or CIN.

☐ 131 The majority of cases lie in the transformation zone.

☐ 132 Isolated AIS high in the endocervical canal is uncommon in young women.

In vaginal intraepithelial neoplasia (VAIN)

☐ 133 10% of women are under 40 years of age.

☐ 134 Over 50% of patients are asymptomatic.

☐ 135 The recurrence rate may be as high as 40%.

In endometrial hyperplasia

☐ 136 Atypical hyperplasia is the only form with a significant risk of progression to malignancy.

☐ 137 A coexistent carcinoma may be found in 5–10% of patients with atypical hyperplasia.

☐ 138 Risk of progression of cystic hyperplasia is < 5%.

☐ 139 Cystic hyperplasia may be managed on the basis of recurrent symptoms.

Regarding vulval cancer

☐ 140 The majority of cases are squamous cell.

☐ 141 The risk of progression of VIN to vulval cancer is 25%.

☐ 142 The risk of progression of VIN is higher in multifocal compared to unifocal disease.

☐ 143 Paget's disease is associated with conconutant genital tract malignancy in 40% of cases.

☐ 144 The risk of malignant transformation of lichen sclerosus is 10%.

With regard to the treatment of vulval cancer

☐ 145 Stage II lesions have a high risk of groin-node metastasis.

☐ 146 Lateralised type-1 and -2 tumours rarely involve groin nodes.

☐ 147 Stage I lateralised lesions should be treated with radical vulvectomy and bilateral lymphadenectomy.

☐ 148 The groin nodes should always be removed.

☐ 149 Younger women have a higher incidence of nodal disease.

Features associated with intrauterine exposure to diethylstilboestrol are

☐ 150 Cervical cockscomb.

☐ 151 Vaginal adenosis.

☐ 152 Clear-cell adenocarcinoma.

☐ 153 CIN. -

Krukenberg tumours

☐ 154 Occur via coelomic spread.

☐ 155 Are sarcomas.

☐ 156 Secrete estrogen.

☐ 157 Secrete gastrin.

☐ 158 Contain signet cells.

Which of the following statements regarding chemotherapy is/are true

- [ ] 159 Doxorubicin (Adriamycin) causes cardiac myopathy.
- [ ] 160 Methotrexate causes haemorrhagic cystitis.
- [ ] 161 Vincristine cause peripheral neuropathy.
- [ ] 162 Cisplatin causes ototoxity.

The following tumours are of germ-cell origin

- [ ] 163 Yolksac tumours.
- [ ] 164 Brenner tumour.
- [ ] 165 Endometriod tumour.
- [ ] 166 Embryonal-cell tumour.
- [ ] 167 Teratoma.

Serous cystadenocarcinoma

- [ ] 168 Is the commonest malignant ovarian tumour.
- [ ] 169 Often contains psammoma bodies.
- [ ] 170 Is bilateral in less than 20% of cases.
- [ ] 171 Presents as stage III disease in 50% of cases.

In 5α-reductase deficiency

- [ ] 172 It occurs as a result of a mutation in the short arm of the Y chromosome.
- [ ] 173 It is associated with virilisation at puberty.
- [ ] 174 Testosterone production occurs normally from the testes.
- [ ] 175 Anti-Mullerian hormone production is deficient.
- [ ] 176 Affected individuals have ambiguous genitalia.

The following reduce the risk of wound dehiscence

- [ ] 177 Tension sutures.
- [ ] 178 Mass closure technique.
- [ ] 179 Prophylactic antibiotics.
- [ ] 180 Polyglycolic sutures.

The ureter

- [ ] 181 Is retroperitoneal in its abdominal course.
- [ ] 182 Passes along the posterior medial aspect of the psoas major.
- [ ] 183 Is crossed inferiorly by the uterine artery.
- [ ] 184 Enters the bladder at the dome.
- [ ] 185 Is crossed by ovarian vessels.

Concerning innervation of the bladder and the urethra

- [ ] 186 The main supply is sympathetic.
- [ ] 187 Cell bodies of the sympathetic supply arise from S2–S4.
- [ ] 188 The parasympathetic supply originates from T10–L2.
- [ ] 189 Parasympathetic effects are mediated by α- and β-receptors.
- [ ] 190 Pelvic splanchnic nerves supply the rhabdosphincter.

Regarding peritoneal closure

- [ ] 191 Non-closure of the peritoneum is associated with increased febrile morbidity.
- [ ] 192 Peritoneal closure at Caesarean section increases the risk of bladder adhesions.
- [ ] 193 Closure of the peritoneum after vaginal surgery is recommended.
- [ ] 194 Use of postoperative analgesia is reduced if the peritoneum is not closed.
- [ ] 195 Non-closure of the peritoneum is associated with a quicker return of bowel activity.

Regarding a simple unilateral ovarian cyst less than 5 cm in diameter with a normal CA125 in a postmenopausal woman

- [ ] 196 It can be managed conservatively.
- [ ] 197 Gives a risk of malignancy of approximately 10%.
- [ ] 198 Cytological examination of aspirated cyst fluid is a useful test.
- [ ] 199 50% resolve spontaneously within 3 months.

In cases of ectopic pregnancy

☐ 200 In the confidential enquiry into maternal deaths ectopic pregnancy remains a major cause of death in the first trimester.

☐ 201 A β-HCG rise of 66% in 48 hours suggests an ectopic pregnancy rather than intrauterine pregnancy.

☐ 202 The serum progesterone level distinguishes well between intrauterine and ectopic pregnancies.

☐ 203 Diagnostic laparoscopy has a false-positive rate of 5%.

☐ 204 A serum progesterone value of > 25 ng/ml suggests an ectopic pregnancy.

In endometriosis

☐ 205 The incidence has a peak prevalence between the ages of 20 and 35 years of age.

☐ 206 The risk is increased sevenfold if there is an affected first-degree relative.

☐ 207 It is more common in dizygotic than monozygotic twins.

☐ 208 The commonest presenting symptom is pelvic pain.

☐ 209 Dyspareunia is reported in over 50% of cases.

Side-effects of danazol include

☐ 210 Acne.

☐ 211 Cholestatic jaundice.

☐ 212 Hirsutism.

☐ 213 Irreversible deepening of the voice.

☐ 214 Thrombocytopenia.

Gestrinone

☐ 215 Acts via binding to progesterone receptors.

☐ 216 Exerts antiestrogenic activity via binding to estrogen receptors.

☐ 217 Has no effect on basal gonadotrophin levels.

☐ 218 70% of patients are amenorrhoeic within 3 months.

☐ 219 Reduces sex-hormone-binding globulin levels.

Risk factors for endometrial carcinoma include

☐ 220 Early menopause.

☐ 221 Obesity.

☐ 222 Nulliparity.

☐ 223 Smoking.

☐ 224 Combined oral contraceptive pill.

Factors that increase the risk of failed termination of pregnancy include

☐ 225 Nulliparity.

☐ 226 Termination at less than 6 weeks' gestation.

☐ 227 Acute retroversion of the uterus.

☐ 228 Uterine abnormalities.

☐ 229 Uterine fibroids.

Regarding emergency contraception

☐ 230 The copper IUD should not be fitted more than 5 days after the first act of unprotected intercourse.

☐ 231 The copper IUD has spermicidal activity.

☐ 232 The copper IUD prevents implantation.

☐ 233 Is less effective than the levonorgestrel-only method.

☐ 234 Is contraindicated in a nulliparous woman.

Regarding the use of progesterone-only emergency contraception

☐ 235 The overall pregnancy rate after use is < 0.5%.

☐ 236 Can only be used once during one cycle.

☐ 237 It is contraindicated in a woman with a past history of an ectopic pregnancy.

☐ 238 It is contraindicated in patients with a history of deep-vein thrombosis.

Urinary tract infections

- [ ] 239 Are strongly associated with the use of diaphragms.
- [ ] 240 Are more common in secretors of histoblood group antigens.
- [ ] 241 *Escherichia coli* is the commonest community-acquired pathogen.
- [ ] 242 Is reported in 5% of up to 1 yr old female children.
- [ ] 243 In school-aged children, it is commoner in girls than boys.

The following are normal parameters of bladder function

- [ ] 244 Residual urine < 100 ml.
- [ ] 245 A peak flow rate on voiding of more than 25 ml/s for a voided volume of 150 ml.
- [ ] 246 A detrusor-pressure rise on voiding of more than 50 cmH_2O.
- [ ] 247 A detrusor-pressure rise of less than 15 cmH_2O on filling the bladder to 500 ml.
- [ ] 248 First desire to void at over 400 ml.

Regarding detrusor overactivity

- [ ] 249 Cystoscopy is a useful diagnostic tool.
- [ ] 250 Patients have an increased bladder wall thickness compared to those with urodynamic stress incontinence.
- [ ] 251 The majority of cases in women are due to bladder-neck obstruction.
- [ ] 252 There is a good relationship between symptoms and urodynamic findings.
- [ ] 253 It is seen more commonly in those with neuropathic personality traits.

Risk factors for ectopic pregnancy include

- [ ] 254 Smoking.
- [ ] 255 Salpingitis isthmica nodosa.
- [ ] 256 Diethylstilbestrol.
- [ ] 257 Luteal-phase defects.

Causes of primary amenorrhoea in a girl with normal external genitalia include

- [ ] 258 Kallman's syndrome.
- [ ] 259 Turner's syndrome.
- [ ] 260 Congenital adrenal hyperplasia.
- [ ] 261 Craniopharyngioma.

In gestational trophoblastic disease

- [ ] 262 Complete moles are usually androgenetic in origin.
- [ ] 263 Partial moles are usually triploid.
- [ ] 264 Partial moles do not transform into choriocarcinomas.
- [ ] 265 An embryo is usually present with a partial mole.
- [ ] 266 Heterozygous complete moles are more common than homozygous moles.

Regarding intraoperative complications

- [ ] 267 The risk of bowel injury at laparoscopic surgery is 1%.
- [ ] 268 Bowel damage during laparoscopy more commonly involves the small bowel.
- [ ] 269 Non-absorbable sutures should be used to repair bladder perforations.
- [ ] 270 Insertion of a Verrey's needle into the bladder requires catheterisation for 5–7 days.
- [ ] 271 The risk of ureteric injury is lowest in laparoscopic versus vaginal and abdominal surgery.

Regarding the following contraceptive methods

- [ ] 272 After stopping the combined pill, 60% of women will ovulate by their third cycle.
- [ ] 273 5% of women will be amenorrhoeic 6 months after stopping the combined pill.
- [ ] 274 Following the final injection of depot medroxy-progesterone, ovulation returns after 4–5 months.
- [ ] 275 Women with a low body mass index are at increased risk of 'post-pill' amenorrhoea.

The clinical staging of cervical cancer includes

☐ 276 Cystoscopy.

☐ 277 Proctoscopy.

☐ 278 Laparoscopy.

☐ 279 Chest X-ray.

☐ 280 Cervical biopsy.

In invasive carcinoma of the cervix

☐ 281 In stage IB tumours, size has little relevance to the 5-year survival rate.

☐ 282 In stage IIB disease, there is extension of tumour from the cervix into the lower third of the vagina.

☐ 283 Barrel-shaped endocervical lesions have a worse prognosis than cervical cancers of a similar stage.

☐ 284 Stage for stage, adenocarcinoma of the cervix has a poorer survival rate than squamous lesions.

☐ 285 Pelvic exenteration is contraindicated if there is a central recurrence after radiotherapy.

In ovarian cancer

☐ 286 30% of women have metastasis by the time of presentation.

☐ 287 Mucinous and endometrioid carcinomas are more likely to be associated with an earlier stage and lower grade than serous cystadenocarcinomas.

☐ 288 The tumour marker CA125 is only associated with mucinous tumours.

☐ 289 The histological type, rather than clinical extent of the tumour, is more important in determining prognosis.

☐ 290 Pleural effusion indicates as stage IV disease.

Bacterial vaginosis

☐ 291 Is commoner in White than Black women.

☐ 292 Is not seen in virgins or lesbians.

☐ 293 Clue cells are seen.

☐ 294 The pH of vaginal discharge is less than 4.5.

☐ 295 Is the commonest cause of vaginal discharge in women of child-bearing age.

In gonorrhoea

☐ 296 50% of women with gonorrhoea have concomitant chlamydial infection.

☐ 297 The incubation period is between 2 and 3 months.

☐ 298 *Neisseria gonorrhoea* is a Gram-positive diplococcus.

☐ 299 Diagnosis can be made on the presence of positive serology.

☐ 300 At least 50% of infected women are asymptomatic.

Risk factors associated with increasing the need for chemotherapy following evacuation of a hydatiform mole are

☐ 301 Younger age.

☐ 302 Pre-evacuation βHCG > 100,000 IU/l.

☐ 303 Gestational age > uterine size.

☐ 304 Use of oral contraceptives prior to evacuation.

☐ 305 Bilateral cystic ovarian enlargement.

With regard to endometrioid carcinoma

☐ 306 They account for 10% of all ovarian tumours.

☐ 307 They are accompanied by ovarian or pelvic endometriosis in up to 42% of cases.

☐ 308 15% are associated with endometrial carcinoma.

☐ 309 20% are seen in continuity with recognisable endometriosis.

With regard to borderline tumours of the ovary

☐ 310 10% of all epithelial tumours are borderline.

☐ 311 They are most commonly serous in type.

☐ 312 DNA ploidy is the most important prognostic factor.

☐ 313 The 5-year survival rate for mucinous borderline tumours is better than for serous tumours.

☐ 314 The majority are confined to the ovary.

Uterine leiomyosarcoma

☐ 315 Is the commonest sarcoma of the uterus.

☐ 316 20% arise from a fibroid.

☐ 317 The majority of patients are nulliparous.

☐ 318 Is more common in Afro-Caribbean women.

☐ 319 20% of cases have vascular invasion at the time of presentation.

Paper 2

Obstetrics

Indicate your answers with a T (True) or F (False) in the box provided. The answers for this section start on page 239.

Regarding obstetric cholestasis

☐ 1 Family studies suggest an autosomal-recessive mode of inheritance.

☐ 2 The risk of stillbirth is related to a deterioration in serum transaminases.

☐ 3 Doppler studies have been shown to be useful in predicting fetal risk.

☐ 4 Ursodeoxycholic acid use is associated with an improvement in total bile acids and liver enzymes.

Pathological adherence of the placenta is associated with

☐ 5 Bicornuate uterus.

☐ 6 Fetal distress in labour.

☐ 7 Placenta praevia.

☐ 8 Previous Caesarean section.

☐ 9 Submucosal myomas.

Fetal alcohol syndrome is associated with

☐ 10 Chromosomal abnormalities.

☐ 11 Epicanthic folds.

☐ 12 Spina bifida.

☐ 13 Macrosomia.

☐ 14 Renal abnormalities.

Idiopathic thrombocytopenic purpura (ITP)

☐ 15 Is commonly complicated by postpartum haemorrhage.

☐ 16 Is associated with an increased risk of perinatal mortality.

☐ 17 Is confirmed by increased numbers of metamyelocytes in the bone marrow.

☐ 18 Is an autoimmune disease.

The following vessels carry oxygenated blood in the fetus

☐ 19 Umbilical artery.

☐ 20 Ductus venosus.

☐ 21 Inferior vena cava as it enters the right atrium.

☐ 22 Carotid artery.

☐ 23 Umbilical vein.

A raised maternal serum AFP level at 16 weeks' gestation may be associated with

☐ 24 Threatened abortion.

☐ 25 Aneuploidy.

☐ 26 Molar pregnancy.

☐ 27 Turner's syndrome.

☐ 28 Down's syndrome.

Routine second-trimester anomaly scanning in the UK

☐ 29 Detects most cases of neural tube defects.

☐ 30 Detects most cases of congenital heart defects.

☐ 31 Detects most cases of trisomy 21

☐ 32 Detects most cases of cerebral palsy.

☐ 33 Detects most cases of major renal abnormality.

Neonatal jaundice is associated with

☐ 34 Galactosaemia.

☐ 35 Sickle-cell disease.

☐ 36 Blood group incompatibility.

☐ 37 Hypothyroidism.

☐ 38 Phenylketonuria.

Cytomegalovirus in pregnancy may be

☐ 39 Acquired from only primary (not secondary) maternal infection.

☐ 40 Always presents in the fetus within the first 24 hours after birth.

☐ 41 The highest risk of transmission to the fetus is when infection occurs during the second trimester.

☐ 42 Is commoner in lower socioeconomic groups.

☐ 43 Is the commonest congenital infection in the UK.

Face presentation

☐ 44 Occurs in 1:500 births.

☐ 45 The mentoposterior position is more favourable for vaginal delivery than the mentoanterior position.

☐ 46 Presents the sub-mentobregmatic diameter to the pelvic brim.

☐ 47 Is associated with anencephaly.

☐ 48 Is associated with prematurity.

Regarding iron supplementation in pregnancy

☐ 49 In women with a healthy diet, routine iron supplementation improves pregnancy outcome.

☐ 50 Ferrous sulphate results in less gastrointestinal complications than ferrous gluconate.

☐ 51 Parenteral iron causes the same haematological response as oral iron.

☐ 52 A higher haemoglobin level reduces the risk of postpartum haemorrhage.

☐ 53 It reduces the risk of antepartum haemorrhage.

The following disorders are correctly associated with the mode of inheritance

☐ 54 Congenital adrenal hyperplasia autosomal-dominant.

☐ 55 Tuberous sclerosis autosomal-dominant.

☐ 56 Marfan's syndrome autosomal-recessive.

☐ 57 Gaucher's disease autosomal-recessive.

☐ 58 Familial hypercholesterolaemia autosomal-recessive.

The normal electrocardiogram in pregnancy shows

☐ 59 A loud, third heart sound.

☐ 60 A Q wave in lead III.

☐ 61 A longer PR interval.

☐ 62 An increase in heart rate.

With regards to fetal neural tube defects

☐ 63 The cerebellum is affected in 50% of cases.

☐ 64 The level of the lesion predicts outcome.

☐ 65 A raised acetylcholinesterase level in amniotic fluid is diagnostic. Prognosis with an encaphalocale is intensely related to amount of herniated cerebral tissue.

☐ 66 Limb movement is a good prognostic sign of limb function after delivery.

☐ 67 May be associated with hydrocephalus.

With regard to biophysical assessment of the fetus

☐ 68 A small for gestational age fetus has smaller heart rate accelerations compared with a normal sized fetus of comparable age.

☐ 69 Fetal breathing is decreased by maternal caffeine intake.

☐ 70 At 40 weeks' gestation a normal fetus will spend 28% of its time breathing when it is active.

☐ 71 A biophysical profile is a good assessment of fetal compromise in cases of maternal diabetes.

☐ 72 Fetal breathing movements increase just prior to delivery.

With regard to umbilical artery Doppler scanning

☐ 73 Reduces the incidence of emergency Caesarean sections in high-risk pregnancies.

☐ 74 Is dependent on the angle of insonation.

☐ 75 The resistance index of zero occurs when the end-diastolic velocities are absent or reversed.

☐ 76 Are dimensionless.

Thyroid disease in pregnancy

☐ 77 Hyperthyroidism occurs in 25% of pregnant women.

☐ 78 Hypothyroidism occurs in < 1% of pregnancies.

☐ 79 Thyroid peroxidase antibodies are associated with hypothyroidism.

☐ 80 Thyrotrophin receptor-stimulating antibodies are a risk factor for Graves' disease.

☐ 81 Thyroid peroxidase antibodies in early pregnancy are associated with a 20% chance of postpartum thyroid dysfunction.

Transvaginal ultrasound measurements of cervical length in pregnancy are indicated for

☐ 82 Previous spontaneous vaginal delivery at 14–28 weeks' gestation.

☐ 83 Previous first trimester miscarriage.

☐ 84 Previous LLETZ or cone biopsy for an abnormal smear.

☐ 85 All multiple pregnancies.

☐ 86 Maternal request.

The following hormones in the fetal circulation are predominantly of maternal origin

☐ 87 Estrogen.

☐ 88 Progesterone.

☐ 89 Insulin.

☐ 90 Adrenocorticotrophic hormone.

☐ 91 Thyroid-stimulating hormone.

Obstetric fistulas

☐ 92 Rectovaginal fistulas are more common than vesicovaginal fistulas.

☐ 93 Usually presents the day after delivery.

☐ 94 The methylene blue test may distinguish a small bladder fistula from a ureteric fistula.

☐ 95 Repair should be performed immediately during the postpartum period.

☐ 96 The suprapubic route of repair should be used as it has a better success rate than the vaginal route.

Shoulder dystocia

☐ 97 Occurs in 1 in 1000 deliveries.

☐ 98 Occurs when the bisacromial diameter is greater than the diameter of the pelvic outlet.

☐ 99 Is associated with a long second stage of labour.

☐ 100 The risk of recurrence is 10%.

☐ 101 A fetal weight > 4 kg is strongly predictive of shoulder dystocia.

Concerning the aetiology of pre-eclampsia

☐ 102 The interstitial trophoblast has been shown to be abnormal.

☐ 103 There is a decreased sensitivity to angiotensin II.

☐ 104 There is a three- to fourfold increase in the risk of developing pre-eclampsia if a first-degree relative has been affected.

☐ 105 Placental hypoperfusion occurs due to a decrease in intervillous blood flow.

☐ 106 There is a raised incidence in women who change partners after the birth of their first child.

In pregnancy-induced hypertension

- [ ] 107 The Korotkoff sound IV corresponds most closely with intra-arterial pressure.
- [ ] 108 The commonly used hypertensives, labetolol, methyldopa and nifedipine, all cross the placenta.
- [ ] 109 The use of calcium supplementation reduces the risk of pre-eclampsia.
- [ ] 110 The use of antihypertensives has reduced the incidence of pre-eclampsia and perinatal mortality rates.
- [ ] 111 There is good evidence for the use of low-dose aspirin to reduce the risk of pre-eclampsia.

In hyperemesis gravidarum

- [ ] 112 5% dextrose should be commenced until oral fluids are tolerated.
- [ ] 113 A metabolic acidosis is characteristically seen.
- [ ] 114 Wernicke's encephalopathy is due to vitamin B_{12} deficiency.
- [ ] 115 50% of patients have abnormal liver function tests.
- [ ] 116 An elevated T_4 and low TSH should be corrected with antithyroid medication.

With regard to inflammatory bowel disease in pregnancy

- [ ] 117 Active disease at the time of conception is associated with an increased risk of miscarriage.
- [ ] 118 The risk of preterm delivery is increased if there is active disease during pregnancy.
- [ ] 119 Azathioprine is contraindicated in pregnancy.
- [ ] 120 Active perianal disease at the time of delivery is an indication for Caesarean section.
- [ ] 121 Pregnancy exacerbates symptoms in the majority of cases.

Regional anaesthesia in labour

☐ 122 Local anaesthetics block C-fibres at lower concentrations than Aδ-fibres.

☐ 123 Opioids block C-fibres at lower concentrations than Aδ-fibres.

☐ 124 Spinal doses of local anaesthetic are 10 times the dose required for epidural anaesthesia.

☐ 125 The incidence of dural puncture headaches is 2%.

☐ 126 Epidural analgesia does not increase the need for Caesarean section.

Maternal smoking in pregnancy is associated with

☐ 127 A reduction in fetal blood flow to the brain.

☐ 128 An increased risk of placental abruption.

☐ 129 An increased risk of pre-eclampsia.

☐ 130 A reduction in fetal breathing movements.

☐ 131 An increased risk of fetal hypoglycaemia.

Type-1 diabetes in pregnancy

☐ 132 Complicates 1% of pregnancies.

☐ 133 Diabetic nephropathy increases the risk of fetal growth restriction, and preterm delivery.

☐ 134 Rapid normalisation of blood glucose levels in pregnancy is associated with an improvement in retinopathy.

☐ 135 The risk of macrosomia is related to maternal postprandial glucose levels.

☐ 136 Tight glycaemic control in labour improves fetal outcome.

In type-1 diabetes

☐ 137 The incidence of chromosomal abnormalities is increased.

☐ 138 There is an increased rate of miscarriage.

☐ 139 Anencephaly is more common.

☐ 140 Serial fetal Doppler assessments are of value for assessing fetal wellbeing.

☐ 141 Uterine artery blood flow is affected by diabetic glycaemic control.

HELLP syndrome

- [ ] 142 30% of cases occur during the second trimester.
- [ ] 143 It can only be diagnosed in the presence of hypertension.
- [ ] 144 Coagulation parameters are usually abnormal.
- [ ] 145 Caesarean section may increase transaminase levels.
- [ ] 146 Has a recurrence risk of 5%.

Amniocentesis

- [ ] 147 Sampling failure rate is 5%.
- [ ] 148 Is complicated by chorioamnionitis in 5% of cases.
- [ ] 149 May cause platelet isoimmunisation.
- [ ] 150 Is associated with limb deformities.
- [ ] 151 The culture failure rate is 2%.

The following clinical signs in a newborn lower the Apgar score

- [ ] 152 Pallor.
- [ ] 153 Fetal pulse > 120 beats per minute.
- [ ] 154 Respiration > 30/minute.
- [ ] 155 Absence of a Moro reflex.
- [ ] 156 Irregular respiration.

In monochorionic diamniotic twin pregnancies

- [ ] 157 The twins are monozygotic.
- [ ] 158 The twins may be dizygotic.
- [ ] 159 The presence of arterial anastomoses is protective against twin–twin transfusion.
- [ ] 160 There is an increased incidence of cerebral palsy.
- [ ] 161 Feto-fetal transfusion syndrome complicates 5% of monochorionic pregnancies.

Asymptomatic bacteriuria in pregnancy

- [ ] 162 Is seen in 10% of women.
- [ ] 163 If left untreated will progress to symptomatic infection in > 50% of women.
- [ ] 164 Is associated with preterm delivery.
- [ ] 165 Is associated with low birth weight.
- [ ] 166 Is more common in pregnancy than in the non-pregnant state.

Rubella in pregnancy

- [ ] 167 5% of parous women are non-immune.
- [ ] 168 Is associated with intrauterine growth retardation.
- [ ] 169 Is only associated with congenital deafness if infection is acquired before 16 weeks' gestation.
- [ ] 170 Is associated with microcephaly.
- [ ] 171 Is associated with thrombocytopenia.

Uteroplacental Doppler assessment

- [ ] 172 Is best performed using continuous-wave Doppler.
- [ ] 173 Normal pregnancies show a reduction in the pulsatility index.
- [ ] 174 High-resistance velocity waveforms are seen in pregnancies at high-risk of pre-eclampsia.
- [ ] 175 High-resistance velocity waveforms are seen in pregnancies at high risk of intrauterine growth retardation.
- [ ] 176 Is a good indicator of fetal hypoxia.

Regarding ultrasound in pregnancy

- [ ] 177 The lambda sign distinguishes a monochorionic from dichorionic pregnancy.
- [ ] 178 Routine ultrasound dating will reduce induction rates.
- [ ] 179 Routine screening has poor sensitivity for the detection of cardiac malformations.
- [ ] 180 In spina bifida the lemon sign is more commonly seen after 24 weeks' gestation than the banana sign.

Toxoplasmosis in pregnancy

☐ 181 Is caused by a bacterium.

☐ 182 70% of infants are asymptomatic at birth.

☐ 183 The severity of fetal infection is less the later it occurs in pregnancy.

☐ 184 The absence of fetal IgM excludes infection.

☐ 185 Maternal treatment with spiramycin reduces the risk of fetal infection.

Congenital infection with cytomegalovirus

☐ 186 Affects up to 2% of live births.

☐ 187 Is associated with hydrocephalus.

☐ 188 Is associated with intrauterine growth retardation.

☐ 189 Occurs only with primary maternal infection.

☐ 190 May be confirmed by culture of an infant's urine.

Listeriosis in pregnancy

☐ 191 Is diagnosed by confirmation of positive serology.

☐ 192 Is a water-borne infection.

☐ 193 Is associated with meningoencephalitis in the neonate.

☐ 194 May present as a rash at birth.

☐ 195 Is associated with contamination of the amniotic fluid with meconium.

Parvovirus B19

☐ 196 Is an RNA virus.

☐ 197 Viraemia is seen after 1 week.

☐ 198 The characteristic rash is seen during maximum viraemia.

☐ 199 May cause fetal hydrops.

☐ 200 May be associated with a myocarditis.

In Down's syndrome

☐ 201 The chromosomal abnormality is more likely to be due to translocation rather than a non-dysfunction.

☐ 202 There is an increased risk of translocation with increasing maternal age.

☐ 203 If the child has a trisomy then the risk of having another affected child is 2%.

☐ 204 If the child has a translocation, the risk of having another affected child is higher if the father rather than the mother carries the balanced translocation.

☐ 205 If the child has a translocation, the risk of having another affected child is 10% if the mother carries the balanced translocation.

Appendicitis in pregnancy

☐ 206 The incidence is lower in pregnancy.

☐ 207 The mortality rate is higher in pregnancy.

☐ 208 Conservative treatment is advised if the fetus is under 24 weeks' gestation.

☐ 209 Maternal and fetal mortality rates are very low if perforation has not occurred.

Pancreatitis in pregnancy

☐ 210 Is more common during the third trimester.

☐ 211 Gallstones are present in over 50% of cases.

☐ 212 Should be managed surgically.

☐ 213 The diagnosis can be made with cholangiopancreatography.

☐ 214 Is associated with hyperparathyroidism.

In normal pregnancy the following coagulation factors are increased

- [ ] 215 Factor X.
- [ ] 216 Factor VII.
- [ ] 217 Factor IIa.
- [ ] 218 Factor XII.
- [ ] 219 Plasma fibrinogen.

Fetal hydrops

- [ ] 220 Is due to red-cell isoimmunisation in the majority of cases.
- [ ] 221 Is due to a chromosomal abnormality in the majority of non-immune cases.
- [ ] 222 Amniocentesis should be recommended.
- [ ] 223 The prognosis is worse if there are large pleural effusions.
- [ ] 224 The best prognosis is seen if it occurs in association with fetal arrhythmias.

Congenital cleft lip and palate

- [ ] 225 Is more common as a unilateral than bilateral defect.
- [ ] 226 Is not associated with aneuploidy.
- [ ] 227 Its risk is increased in future pregnancies.
- [ ] 228 Is associated with antiepileptic medication.

Systemic lupus erythematosus in pregnancy

- [ ] 229 There is a decreased risk of flare-up in pregnancy.
- [ ] 230 Is associated with an increased risk of abortion.
- [ ] 231 Anti-Ro antibodies are present in 15% of patients.
- [ ] 232 Anti-Ro antibodies cross the placenta.
- [ ] 233 Cutaneous lupus is seen in 50% of babies of anti-Ro positive mothers.

Rheumatoid arthritis in pregnancy

- [ ] 234 The disease will deteriorate in the majority of women during pregnancy.
- [ ] 235 Symptoms usually improve postpartum.
- [ ] 236 There is an increased rate of miscarriage.
- [ ] 237 Azathioprine is contraindicated.
- [ ] 238 Sulfasalazine is safe in pregnancy.

Peripartum cardiomyopathy

- [ ] 239 Can occur up to six months' postpartum.
- [ ] 240 Is more common in primiparous patients.
- [ ] 241 Is more common in Black women.
- [ ] 242 Requires anticoagulation.
- [ ] 243 Recurrence is common.

The normal haemodynamic changes in pregnancy include

- [ ] 244 An increase in plasma volume, particularly during the third trimester.
- [ ] 245 A decrease in pulse volume.
- [ ] 246 The rise in cardiac output in pregnancy returns to normal in the first 24 hours' postpartum.
- [ ] 247 A diastolic murmur is a common, normal physiological finding.

In the management of labour

- [ ] 248 Engagement of the vertex occurs when the biparietal diameter passes the pelvic outlet.
- [ ] 249 Active management of labour reduces the Caesarean section risk.
- [ ] 250 Oxytocin should not be used if cephalopelvic disproportion is suspected.
- [ ] 251 Amniotomy is associated with an increased risk of instrumental delivery.
- [ ] 252 Two out of three women who have had a previous Caesarean section for cephalopelvic disportion will have a subsequent vaginal delivery.

Anti-D prophylaxis

☐ 253 Should be given to all non-sensitised rhesus-negative women after amniocentesis or chorionic villus sampling (CVS).

☐ 254 Should be given to all non-sensitised Rh D-negative women after a threatened miscarriage.

☐ 255 Sensitisation by undetected fetomaternal haemorrhage occurs in the third trimester in 90% of cases.

☐ 256 Routine administration of 500 IU anti-D should be given to all non-sensitised Rh- negative primigravidas at 28 weeks' and 34 weeks' gestation.

☐ 257 Kleihauer testing should be carried out on any sensitising event after 20 weeks' gestation.

In a woman with prosthetic heart valves

☐ 258 There is a high risk of bacterial endocarditis during delivery.

☐ 259 Usually have a decreased cardiac reserve.

☐ 260 Heparin use for anticoagulation is associated with a higher rate of thromboembolic complications.

☐ 261 Oxytocin is contraindicated in labour.

☐ 262 The risk of teratogenicity from warfarin is greatest at 9–12 weeks' gestation.

The small for gestational age (SGA) fetus

☐ 263 An amniotic fluid index of < 0.5 cm is associated with an increased risk of an Apgar score < 7 at five minutes.

☐ 264 70% of fetuses with an abdominal circumference and estimated fetal weight < 5th centile have chromosomal defects.

☐ 265 20% of normally formed stillbirths are small for gestational age.

☐ 266 The ratio of head to abdominal circumference is more accurate than abdominal circumference or estimated fetal weight (EFW) alone in predicting the SGA fetus.

☐ 267 Is associated with the development of type-2 diabetes in adult life.

Chickenpox in pregnancy

- [ ] 268 The incubation period is 5–10 days.
- [ ] 269 Shingles before 20 weeks' gestation has a 1% risk of fetal abnormality.
- [ ] 270 Varicella immunoglobulin given to the mother within the first 24 hours of contact with chickenpox prevents intrauterine infection.
- [ ] 271 Congenital varicella may be detected on a second-trimester anomaly scan.

Amniotic fluid

- [ ] 272 The 15th and 95th centiles for the amniotic fluid index are 5–15 cm.
- [ ] 273 Is reduced in upper gastrointestinal obstruction.
- [ ] 274 Is reduced in bilateral uropathy.
- [ ] 275 Is reduced in fetuses with neural tube defects.
- [ ] 276 Is increased in maternal diabetes.

In fetal red-cell alloimmunisation

- [ ] 277 The indirect Coombs' test can detect the presence of antibodies in serum.
- [ ] 278 Maternal serum anti-D below 4 IU/ml is not associated with severe fetal anaemia.
- [ ] 279 There is an increase in Doppler blood-flow velocity in fetal vessels in severe anaemia.
- [ ] 280 Severe fetal anaemia is always characterised by poor fetal movements and hydrops.
- [ ] 281 The survival rate of a hydropic fetus after intrauterine transfusion is approximately 50%.

Postpartum haemorrhage

☐ 282 May be associated with platelet deficiency.

☐ 283 Fresh-frozen plasma should ideally be given with every 2 units of blood.

☐ 284 Hyperkalaemia may be a complication of blood transfusion.

☐ 285 The blood volume should be restored until the central venous pressure is 5 cmH$_2$O.

☐ 286 Cryoprecipitate should be given if the fibrinogen level is less than 10 g/dl.

Herpes gestation in pregnancy

☐ 287 Is due to a herpesvirus.

☐ 288 Diagnosis is made on the serology results.

☐ 289 Usually recurs in subsequent pregnancies.

☐ 290 Is associated with low birth weight and preterm delivery.

☐ 291 Systemic steroids should be withheld until after delivery.

HIV in pregnancy

☐ 292 Without intervention the mother-to-child transmission rate is up to 30%.

☐ 293 Breastfeeding doubles the risk of mother child transmission (CT).

☐ 294 There is an increased risk of complications at Caesarean section.

☐ 295 A viral load < 2000 copies/ml is not associated with fetal infection.

☐ 296 Antiretroviral treatment should be commenced as soon as the diagnosis is known.

Regarding the death of one twin in a monochorionic twin pregnancy

☐ 297 It is associated with a 25% risk of death in the surviving twin.

☐ 298 It is associated with a 50% risk of cerebral damage in the surviving twin.

☐ 299 The appearance of porencephaly in the surviving twin indicates severe brain damage.

☐ 300 Delivery should be delayed as long as possible until there is structural evidence of brain damage.

☐ 301 There is no risk of fetal brain damage in the surviving twin of a dichorionic twin pregnancy.

In any set of observations

☐ 302 The mean is less than the mode.

☐ 303 Half the observations are less than the median.

☐ 304 If the data is skewed to the right, the median is less than the mean.

☐ 305 The mode is always the most frequently occurring value.

☐ 306 The variance is the square root of the standard deviation.

Urine cytology was studied in 100 women with haematuria to assess the accuracy of urine cytology in the detection of bladder cancer. In this group, 20 women had positive cytology. At the end of the study 10 women had confirmed bladder cancers, but only 5 had positive cytology. With regard to urine cytology for the detection of bladder cancer

☐ 307 The sensitivity of the test is 50%.

☐ 308 The specificity of the test is 10%.

☐ 309 The negative predictive value is 5%.

☐ 310 The positive predictive value is 25%.

Essays

Gynaecological essays

Essay 1

A 34-year-old, nulliparous woman has been found to have a pelvic mass. Ultrasound scan confirmed the presence of multiple uterine fibroids.

Critically appraise your management.

Essay tips

The key words in this question are:

- 34-year-old, nulliparous
- pelvic mass – the nature of it (multiple uterine fibroids), confirmed by ultrasound scan
- critically appraise
- management.

34-year-old, nulliparous

Preservation of fertility may be an issue as she is 34 years of age and nulliparous. Did she try to become pregnant and what are her wishes? What is her past gynaecological history, and social history – partner, etc?

Pelvic mass – the nature of it (multiple fibroids in this case) confirmed by ultrasound scan

You want to know the size of the mass and whether she has any associated symptoms such as pain, menstrual disorders, urinary and/or bowel symptoms, and any adverse effects on her quality of life – it's always worthwhile mentioning the latter in women with benign gynaecological conditions.

Multiple fibroids

This question aims to explore your knowledge of uterine fibroids and their management in different clinical circumstances. Your essay should therefore focus on uterine fibroids in the particular patient described, not on how to investigate/manage a pelvic mass in general.

The diagram is to aid your recall of the factors commonly associated with fibroids.

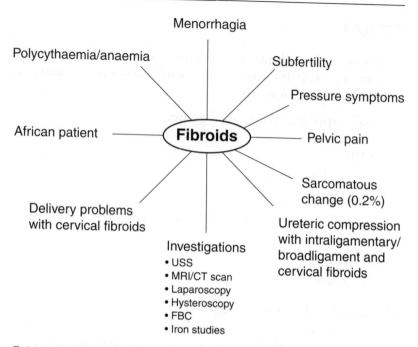

Menorrhagia

Polycythaemia/anaemia

Subfertility

Pressure symptoms

African patient — **Fibroids** — Pelvic pain

Sarcomatous change (0.2%)

Delivery problems with cervical fibroids

Ureteric compression with intraligamentary/ broadligament and cervical fibroids

Investigations
- USS
- MRI/CT scan
- Laparoscopy
- Hysteroscopy
- FBC
- Iron studies

Critically appraise

Mention the pros and cons of any management options you propose or advocate for this particular case. You may start the sentence with, 'Depending on..., but *I* would...; however, this may cause...or...lead to...'.

Management

Management questions are about the history, examination, investigations and treatment options. The treatment may be expectant; pharmacological, surgical or alternative medical methods; and involve follow-up.

Treatment options
These could be:

- **None**:
  - for a small mass and in an asymptomatic patient.

- **Non-hormonal**:
  - tranexamic acid: prescribe mefenamic acid in the case of a small mass/a woman who wishes to conceive/for mainly menstrual problems.

- **Hormonal**:
  - oral contraceptive pill if she has menstrual problems and needs contraception.
  - GnRH-analogues: a three-month course may reduce the size of fibroids by up to 40–60%. Their main drawbacks include: expense; regrowth of fibroids after withdrawal of treatment; limited duration of use because of skeletal effects; and menopausal side-effects. They may be used prior to myomectomy. (Note that the efficacy of GnRH-analogues in reducing the size of uterine fibroids is better when used to treat a single large fibroid than multiple small fibroids.)
  - danazol has significant androgenic side-effects.

- **Surgical**:
  - laparoscopy or hysteroscopy: subserous versus submucous fibroids can be managed in this way. Mention the: potential hazards of both; expense of instruments; the need for advanced surgical training; and the risk of recurrence.
  - open myomectomy: may be associated with severe haemorrhage. Intramyoma injection of vasopressin may be used to reduce blood loss together with meticulous attention to haemostasis. There is a small but finite risk of conversion to hysterectomy. This is a common treatment for heavy menstrual loss but may be unacceptable to this particular woman.

The essay itself

The clinical challenge in the management of uterine fibroids in a nulliparous, reproductive-age woman centres around the preservation of child-bearing capabilities and the potential complications of interventions on the one hand, and the effective relief or elimination of symptoms on the other.

History

One would explore her menstrual history to subjectively establish the quantity of menstrual loss (number of sanitary towels/tampons required, clots, flooding, anaemia, etc), subfertility, pelvic pain, urinary and or bowel symptoms, as well as their impact on her life (eg house-bound during periods).

Examination

A full general physical examination should be performed, looking for signs of anaemia followed by an abdominal examination to assess the size and mobility of the fibroid mass. The findings may determine the type of skin incision if surgery is subsequently embarked on. A speculum vaginal examination to inspect the cervix may be unsuccessful as the position of the cervix is frequently distorted in these cases. Bimanual pelvic examination is required to confirm the size and mobility of the uterus. The scan would have excluded ovarian pathology.

Investigations

These should include a full blood count as well as iron studies if there is anaemia. An intravenous urogram is very rarely required to exclude ureteric obstruction in cases of broad ligament, cervical or very large fibroids.

Treatment

This depends on the presenting signs and symptoms, and the wishes and expectations of the patient.

- A completely asymptomatic patient can be managed expectantly.
- If anaemia is present, this should be corrected with iron therapy or blood transfusion, depending on the degree of anaemia.
- Tranexamic acid and/or mefenamic acid may be considered for a woman with small fibroids and minimal menstrual problems.

- GnRH-analogues improve haemoglobin levels. A three-months' course may shrink fibroids by as much as 40–60%, which might make future myomectomy easier. However, these drugs are expensive and cause vasomotor/menopausal symptoms. Some clinicians also report a loss of the plane of cleavage between the fibroid and its capsule, making enucleation of the fibroids difficult even though they have been reduced in size.
- The oral contraceptive pill is a cost-effective alternative.
- Danazol is also potentially effective but is not well tolerated due to its androgenic side-effects.
- If subfertility is a problem and the fibroids are the only identifiable cause, myomectomy may be considered, either hysteroscopically for submucous fibroids or laparoscopically for subserous and pedunculated fibroids. However, the equipment required for these options is expensive and advanced surgical training is needed to acquire the relevant expertise.
- Hysterosalpingography (HSG)/hysterosalpingo-contrast-sonography (HyCoSy) may be required to evaluate intracavity distortion before hysteroscopic surgery.
- Open myomectomy carries the additional risk of major surgery and the risk of hysterectomy. Good haemostasis and vasopressin intraoperatively may help to prevent this.
- Subtotal or total hysterectomy is the definitive treatment for fibroids. However, it is unlikely to be acceptable to this particular woman unless her condition is disabling, eg intractable vaginal bleeding or a degenerating fibroid.
- Follow-ups should be arranged at sensible intervals (if she is managed conservatively).

Other suggestions

Uterine artery embolisation is another option open to this woman. This requires an interventional radiologist input. The procedure is effective in over 60% of cases. There is a 1–2% risk of loss of ovarian function. This is more common in women over 40 years of age and those with a higher baseline FSH level. There is also scanty data on subsequent reproductive performance of the uterus after embolisation. At present it is not considered suitable for women intending to embark on a pregnancy in future.

Essay 2

A 42-year-old multiparous woman presents with a six-month history of intermenstrual bleeding (IMB).

Justify your investigations.

Essay tips

The key words in this question are:

- 42 years of age
- multiparous
- six months
- justify
- investigations.

42 years of age

First, determine her smear history. Second, find out if she has coexistent gynaecological problems, for example fibroids or heavy menstrual loss. Third, she is over 40 years of age and, according to RCOG guidelines, hysteroscopy and endometrial biopsy are recommended diagnostic steps. Medical conditions may be present in women of this age and they will have a direct impact on treatment. So the history should explore other systems including problems like diabetes and thyroid dysfunction.

Multiparous

Ask about her past obstetric history, sexual contacts (sexually transmitted diseases?), social history and contraception. Does she feel her family is now complete?

Six months

A time is given in the question that points towards the need to carefully evaluate her cycle, eg length, presence of postcoital bleeding, a previous episode of IMB and how was it treated? Has she had colposcopy or hormone treatment in the past? How heavy is her IMB, and does she have any associated pain?

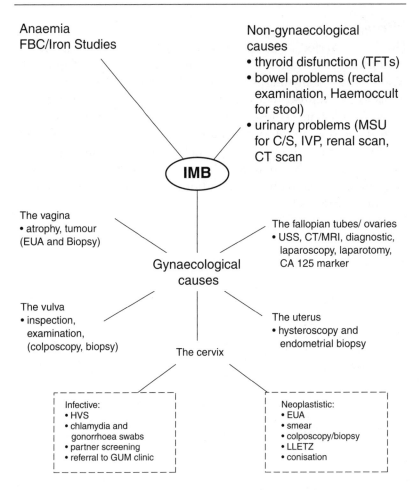

Anaemia
FBC/Iron Studies

Non-gynaecological causes
• thyroid disfunction (TFTs)
• bowel problems (rectal examination, Haemoccult for stool)
• urinary problems (MSU for C/S, IVP, renal scan, CT scan

IMB

The vagina
• atrophy, tumour (EUA and Biopsy)

The fallopian tubes/ ovaries
• USS, CT/MRI, diagnostic, laparoscopy, laparotomy, CA 125 marker

Gynaecological causes

The vulva
• inspection, examination, (colposcopy, biopsy)

The uterus
• hysteroscopy and endometrial biopsy

The cervix

Infective:
• HVS
• chlamydia and gonorrhoea swabs
• partner screening
• referral to GUM clinic

Neoplastistic:
• EUA
• smear
• colposcopy/biopsy
• LLETZ
• conisation

In these types of question, the history and examination determine the appropriate investigations. As outlined, the causes of her IMB might be gynaecological or non-gynaecological. The latter should be mentioned, and the list at the top of the figure can be effectively summarised in three or four concise sentences.

Justify

Why would you do what, and on the grounds of what evidence? If English is not your first language the word 'because' is very useful in justifying your actions and options. Alternatively, you could use 'therefore' or 'that's why'. In other words, give the reasons why you would do/request a specific test.

Investigations

Don't be carried away into discussing the management of the patient. This is time-consuming, and for this type of question won't earn you any marks. Example: If a frank cervical carcinoma is suspected, representative biopsies should be taken and an examination under anaesthesia performed, including cystoscopy and rectosigmoidoscopy. Additional tests will include chest X-ray, U&E and IVP (intravenous pyelogram), helping to determine the extent of the disease. No marks will be awarded for the sentence 'Wertheim's hysterectomy or radiotherapy are the two possible treatment options'!

The essay itself

Start by defining IMB (sometimes there is a mark for this). Intermenstrual bleeding (IMB) describes bleeding between periods.

It would be unhelpful to dwell on the patient's history since the question has already provided the relevant information. Outline the key and relevant aspects of the patient's history in one or two sentences.

The question is really about the characteristics and reliability of the tests used in the investigation of IMB. More importantly, the majority of these cases are secondary to the transient but physiological fall in estradiol levels after ovulation, prior to the amplified output by the corpus luteum. Alternatively, there may be dysfunctional uterine bleeding of the anovulatory type, which is common in this age group. You should focus your answer on the role, sensitivities, specificities, positive and negative predictive values of the tests, and describe the relevant clinical indications for these tests in your answer.

History

The history should include details of: the bleeding – how heavy it is, and when it occurs in relation to her cycle; drug use – for instance, tamoxifen, contraception (eg Depo-Provera); and the patient's past gynaecological, medical and surgical history. Cycle length is also relevant as well as the occurrence of vasomotor symptoms.

Examination

Comment briefly on the general and gynaecological examination, including signs of anaemia, or goitre, tachycardia and/or exophthalmos pointing toward thyroid dysfunction. Therefore a full blood count and thyroid function test form part of the basic investigations.

Logically, a gynaecological examination should be performed in the following order: examination of the vulva; speculum examination of the vagina and cervix; and bimanual examination to evaluate the uterus and adnexae.

The vulva and vagina should be thoroughly inspected and in the presence of vulval pain and pruritus, colposcopy and targeted biopsies should be performed.

At speculum examination, the cervix should be visualised, a smear taken as well as high vaginal and endocervical swabs for chlamydia and other sexually transmitted pathogens. Fibroids or polyps may be present, which can be further evaluated by transvaginal ultrasound (TVS) including saline-diffusion sonography (to improve diagnostic accuracy and to detect endometrial polyps). An endometrial Pipelle biopsy should be obtained to exclude endometrial hyperplasia or malignancy, especially if there are no facilities for hysteroscopy in the out-patients department. Colposcopy should be performed and a biopsy taken if the cervix appears suspicious or if the patient has a history of abnormal smears.

Doppler studies of the ovarian vessels and endometrium may be considered if there are any suspicious sonographic features in these organs. Hysteroscopy and directed biopsy is the investigation of choice over the traditional D&C (dilatation and curettage) as the latter is blind and samples less than 50% of the cavity and misses polyps.

In any case, hysteroscopy should be performed and an endometrial biopsy taken as well as more advanced tests, eg CT/MRI, since this patient is over 40 years of age. If carcinoma of the cervix is diagnosed then the patient should undergo an examination under anaesthesia (EUA) and staging.

Adnexal masses are uncommon causes of IMB. However, if masses are found then further investigations, such as pelvic ultrasound and Doppler scans, CA125 and diagnostic laparoscopy may be necessary.

Extragenital sources of bleeding should be ruled out. If the bleeding is found to originate from the bowel or the renal tract then a mid-stream urine sample should be obtained and a recto- and sigmoidoscopy arranged, as well as cystoscopy. A CT scan or MRI may be added if appropriate.

Essay 3

A 25-year-old, obese woman has noticed excessive hair growth over the past 12 months.

Discuss your further management.

Essay tips

The key words in this question are:

- 25 years of age – obese
- excessive hair growth
- 12 months
- discuss
- management.

25 years of age – obese

This combination of symptoms suggests the diagnosis of polycystic ovarian disease (PCOD). The following diagram highlights the spectrum of clinical disease.

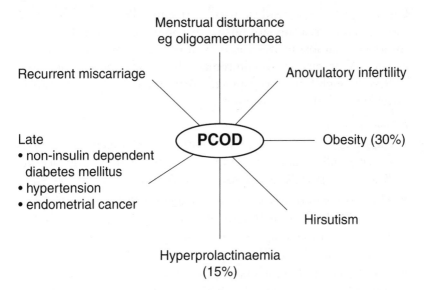

A background history is essential since this is a 'management' question. The points to cover include: menstrual history;

headache; diminished visual field; galactorrhoea; past obstetric history, history of infertility treatment, recurrent miscarriage; family history of gynaecological malignancy; social history, including partner(s), work, drug and alcohol use.

Excessive hair growth

The speed of onset; distribution; signs of virilism, such as temporal balding, deepening of the voice, breast atrophy; and a drug history, eg danazol.

Explore the patient's family history and racial background. Assess the psychological impact of her situation.

Twelve months

A benign aetiology is more likely as her symptoms developed over a 12-month period. However, a comment to the effect that 'malignant tumours of the ovaries or the adrenals should be excluded' demonstrates your clinical astuteness and attention to detail.

Discuss

Discuss' may be considered to be the middle ground between 'justify' and 'critically appraise'. In some ways it involves both. Although it almost invites you to 'waffle', this should be vigorously resisted. Your answers should remain short and concise. The aim is to have enough time and paper to create the different scenarios in order to cover the various points.

Examples

- Mild hirsutism may be treated with the combined oral contraceptive pill. Dianette, which contains cyproterone acetate (CPA), is especially useful for this indication.

- The more severe cases can be managed with a reversed regime using CPA in the first 10 days of each cycle. Pregnancy should be avoided for three months after cessation of treatment because of the long half-life of CPA.

- Psychological support should be considered for patients with severe hirsutism, especially if there is associated psychological morbidity. Cosmetic treatment may be started in the first instance, eg waxing, peeling and electrolysis. The latter may be painful and expensive. Non-hormonal agents such as spirono-lactone may be used, although this requires regular monitoring of serum electrolytes, K^+ in particular, and contraception to prevent potential feminisation of the male fetus.

• Mild', 'moderate', 'severe' and words like 'if', 'in case of', 'however', 'depending on' may be used repeatedly to cover the wide spectrum of clinical presentations.

Management

Answers to 'management' questions should be structured to cover the following key areas: history, examination, investigations, treatment and follow-up. If the question simply asks about the 'treatment' then a structure built around non-hormonal, hormonal, surgical and alternative treatments is recommended. Do not overlook the follow-up.

The essay itself

Hirsutism is most commonly driven by benign aetiological conditions. However, malignant tumours of the ovaries and adrenal glands or Cushing's syndrome should not be overlooked.

History

Polycystic ovarian disease (PCOD) appears to be the likely cause in this case. Therefore a short history should aim to establish the pattern of her menstrual cycles, the presence of headaches, visual field disturbances and galactorrhoea. Her racial background and a family history of hirsutism should be defined. A history of recurrent miscarriage, subfertility treatment and non-insulin-dependent diabetes mellitus should be explored, as well as her social history, including her partner(s). The speed of onset of hirsutism, its distribution and the extent of any psychological effect on the patient should be established. A drug history is also important, for example Danazol can produce androgenic side-effects.

Examination

A full general and gynaecological examination should be performed, paying particular attention to signs of virilism, for example temporal balding, deepening of the voice, breast atrophy and clitoromegaly. Taking a photograph, or alternatively a Ferriman Galway score, can monitor hair distribution and response to therapy. Cushingoid features, like buffalo neck, should be sought. Pelvic examination should focus on adnexal masses, although androgen-secreting ovarian tumours may be too small to palpate. The patient's blood pressure should also be measured.

Investigations

Initial investigations should include a pelvic ultrasound scan and measurement of early- to mid-follicular phase luteinising hormone (LH)/follicle-stimulating hormone (FSH) levels, prolactin, testosterone, dehydroepiandrosterone sulphate (DHEAS), 17-hydroxy-progesterone (17 OH-P), thyroid function and sex hormone-binding globulin (SHBG). A serum testosterone level > 6 nmol/L should prompt a search for an ovarian tumour or adrenal hyperplasia, therefore necessitating a CT scan or MRI. If Cushing's syndrome is suspected, a 24-hour urinary free cortisol level or short dexamethasone test should be ordered. This patient's fasting blood glucose and lipid profiles should also be checked to exclude impaired glucose/lipid metabolism.

Treatment

Weight loss increases SHBG levels and reduces bioavailable testosterone. Mild hirsutism may be treated with the oral contraceptive pill, especially Dianette which contains the anti-androgen cyproterone acetate (CPA). This increases SHBG levels (thereby reducing bioavailable androgens) and also regulates the menstrual cycle.

The more severe cases may be treated with a reversed sequential regime of CPA 50–100 mg. Pregnancy should be avoided for three months after the cessation of treatment because of the long half-life of CPA and the risk of feminisation of a male fetus. This risk also applies to non-hormonal preparations like spironolactone. In addition, patients taking spironolactone should have their electrolyte, especially potassium, levels monitored regularly. A small dose of dexamethasone (0.5 mg) will help to control raised DHEAS levels. Tumours of the ovaries or adrenals should be treated surgically. A psychologist should be involved in cases of severe hirsutism with psychological symptoms, and cosmetic treatment such as waxing, peeling, shaving and electrolysis offered. However, this may be painful and expensive. The patient should be advised that hair growth is likely once treatment is stopped.

Follow-up

Treatment is time-consuming and follow-up should be arranged at appropriate intervals such as six monthly.

Essay 4

Critically appraise the different options available for the surgical treatment of menorrhagia.

Essay tips

The key words in this question are:

- critically appraise
- different options
- available
- surgical treatment
- menorrhagia.

Critically appraise

The pros and cons and evidence base of any surgical option should be addressed. Other associated factors such as patients' morbidity, cosmetic results, pain relief, hospital stay/cost to the National Health Service, equipment and operating time need to be balanced and critically appraised.

Different options

Don't just talk about total abdominal hysterectomy and vaginal hysterectomy. Structure this part of the essay into traditional/newer methods, major surgery/minimal invasive surgery, abdominal/vaginal surgery, etc.

Available

Some procedures may be under evaluation in their developmental stages and only used in research and controlled experimental conditions. Strictly speaking, such procedures are not 'available' for general clinical use. Equally, that a technique or procedure is not used or available in your hospital does not mean that it does not exist! Update your knowledge and familiarise yourself with newer techniques such as laparoscopic-assisted vaginal hysterectomy and the different methods of endometrial ablation.

Surgical treatment

Whenever surgical treatment comes up, remember the sentence: 'Patient selection is vitally important'. Factors like age, fertility needs, past obstetric and gynaecological history, social history and coexistent gynaecological disease need to be considered. The other fundamental consideration in surgical management options is the availability of 'an appropriately trained and experienced surgeon either operating or directly supervising the procedure'. Examiners approve of candidates' demonstration of their knowledge of clinical governance implications. Another approach is to use short sentences that bring the topic into context with the recent CEPOD report.

Menorrhagia

Again don't get carried away with discussing fibroids, endometriosis and so on. Even if your favourite management option is the Mirena coil this is not what the question is asking for. Besides, it is not a surgical option.

The diagram on the next page is useful for a quick review of the subject.

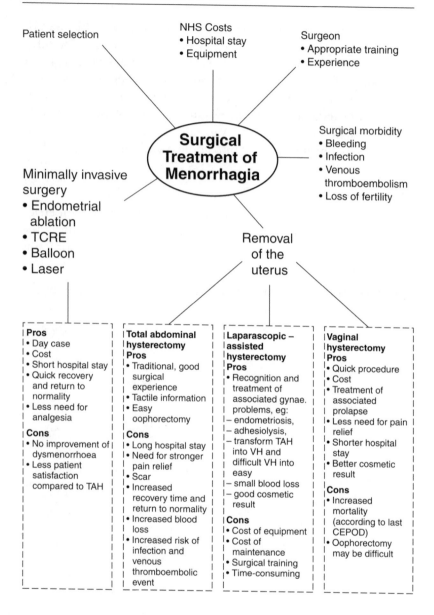

Patient selection

NHS Costs
• Hospital stay
• Equipment

Surgeon
• Appropriate training
• Experience

Surgical Treatment of Menorrhagia

Surgical morbidity
• Bleeding
• Infection
• Venous thromboembolism
• Loss of fertility

Minimally invasive surgery
• Endometrial ablation
• TCRE
• Balloon
• Laser

Removal of the uterus

Pros
• Day case
• Cost
• Short hospital stay
• Quick recovery and return to normality
• Less need for analgesia

Cons
• No improvement of dysmenorrhoea
• Less patient satisfaction compared to TAH

Total abdominal hysterectomy
Pros
• Traditional, good surgical experience
• Tactile information
• Easy oophorectomy

Cons
• Long hospital stay
• Need for stronger pain relief
• Scar
• Increased recovery time and return to normality
• Increased blood loss
• Increased risk of infection and venous thromboembolic event

Laparascopic – assisted hysterectomy
Pros
• Recognition and treatment of associated gynae. problems, eg:
– endometriosis,
– adhesiolysis,
– transform TAH into VH and difficult VH into easy
– small blood loss
– good cosmetic result

Cons
• Cost of equipment
• Cost of maintenance
• Surgical training
• Time-consuming

Vaginal hysterectomy
Pros
• Quick procedure
• Cost
• Treatment of associated prolapse
• Less need for pain relief
• Shorter hospital stay
• Better cosmetic result

Cons
• Increased mortality (according to last CEPOD)
• Oophorectomy may be difficult

The essay itself

The surgical management of menorrhagia has undergone significant changes and modifications in recent years.

Patient selection is vitally important because haemorrhage, infection and thromboembolism may complicate surgical procedures. These complications need to be balanced against the treatment of a benign condition. Therefore the research and development of non-surgical alternative methods of treatment are welcome. Age, future childbearing capability, coexistent medical and gynaecological disease as well as past obstetrics/gynaecological/medical and surgical history all need to be examined carefully as these may affect subsequent patient satisfaction with surgery.

Surgical options

Hysterectomy is the definitive treatment of menorrhagia. Total abdominal hysterectomy (TAH) has the advantage of easy access and good vision of structures like uterus, bladder/bowel and, if needed, affords easy oophorectomy. The patients, however, may incur other intra- or postoperative morbidity including cosmetic effects of a scar – particularly if a midline incision was necessary. Costs to the NHS due to prolonged hospital stays and prolonged pain relief are relevant. The risk of haemorrhage, thromboembolism and infections cannot be ignored. Laparoscopic-assisted vaginal hysterectomy (LAVH) enables a TAH to be transformed into a vaginal hysterectomy (VH), or a difficult VH into an easy one. Although the operating time is prolonged, it compares favourably with VH in terms of patients' recovery, time, reduced pain relief and shorter hospital stay. It is the method of choice in suspected adnexal mass, suspected endometriosis and adhesiolysis.

In addition to the advantages mentioned above, vaginal hysterectomy gives an improved cosmetic result. Oophorectomy can be successfully performed in 95% of patients. Intriguingly, mortality is somewhat higher than with TAH as shown in the last CEPOD report.

The various methods of endometrial resection have been endorsed in the recent past. Endometrial resection is minimally invasive and can be performed as a day-case procedure. However, patient satisfaction and amenorrhoea rate is less than with TAH, and dysmenorrhoea cannot be cured. Risks are intraoperative fluid retention causing pulmonary oedema, coma and death. Haemorrhage, infection and pregnancy complications can occur, and endometrial cancer might be easily overlooked in the future.

Essay 5

Urinary incontinence represents a major health problem for many women.

Justify your diagnostic steps.

Essay tips

The key words are:

- urinary incontinence
- a major health problem for many women
- justify
- diagnostic steps.

Urinary incontinence

The question did not specify that this is urodynamic stress incontinence, detrusor overactivity or a mixed picture. So first divide your essay plan into different forms of incontinence as shown in the figure.

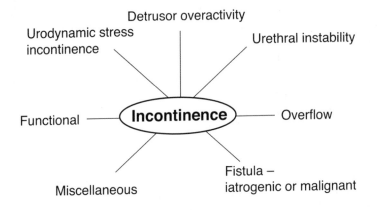

A major health problem for many women

This statement should be assumed to be true and therefore doesn't need to be confirmed (eg written as an 'Introduction' again) or argued (eg 'Though the majority of cases are easily treatable') or extended (eg 'Causes a huge deficit in the health service budgets'). Be careful – this is a trap inviting you to waffle and gain no marks! A statement is a statement! Unless the RCOG asks you to 'Discuss this statement' leave well alone!

Justify

In this particular question 'justify' means: Which test are you going to order, in what circumstances, and why?

Diagnostic steps

Put differently, your pathway to reaching a diagnosis and particularly your 'investigations'. However, before you can justify any investigations you have to take a history and examine the patient. Careful again! Your essay finishes with investigations. No sentences are required about the dry mouth with oxybutynin or the osteitis pubis with the Marshall/Marchetti-Krantz procedure. These are treatment options and side-effects of the same, which haven't been asked for!

Naturally, treatment follows the investigations and diagnostic steps, ie: history, examination, bedside tests and investigations only. It is sensible to start with the least invasive test (eg MSU for culture and sensitivity, or the pad test) and continue to the more invasive/expensive tests, eg videocystourethrography.

History

The points to focus on in the history of any urogynaecology patient include: duration, frequency, urgency, nocturia, and haematuria. Furthermore, the patient's age, occupation (does it involve lifting heavy objects?), chest conditions, constipation, drugs (eg diuretics), drinking habits (eg tea and alcohol), smoking, previous incontinence treatment (surgery) and effects on lifestyle as well as coexistent gynaecological problems have to be explored.
Past obstetric history is also important!

Examination

A full general and gynaecological examination should be performed, including examination of the chest (for chronic cough) and heart (for signs of cardiac failure), abdominal palpation for any masses and a speculum examination to rule out an obvious urinary fistula and vaginal atrophy. A Sim's speculum in the left lateral position is the examination of choice for demonstrating gross stress incontinence and associated cystocele and rectocele.

A pelvic examination is used to check the mobility of the anterior vaginal wall and to detect the presence of masses, eg large fibroids and ovarian masses.

Investigations

Now you may proceed to justify your investigations by introducing different scenarios and applying the tests you think are appropriate.

Examples

- A patient with classical frequency, urgency and dysuria should provide a mid-stream urine sample for culture and sensitivity (C/S) testing.

- A fluid/volume chart is cheap and informative and should be a baseline investigation.

- A pad test is simple and gives some information on the quantity of urine loss.

- If there is an associated haematuria then cytoscopy and an intravenous urogram is mandatory to rule out malignant serious or other underlying pathology.

- Videocystourethrography is a standard investigation, and is particularly useful in patients with previously failed incontinence surgery or vesicoureteric reflux.

- Symptoms pointing towards detrusor overactivity might be best investigated with ambulatory urodynamics, as well as an ultrasound scan to determine the thickness of the bladder wall.

- Flow studies are useful prior to surgery in patients with urodynamic stress incontinence, as a poor flow rate impairs the chance of successful surgery.

The figure on the following page gives a quick reminder.

The essay itself

Appropriate investigations in urogynaecology are largely determined by the information elicited from the history and the examination findings.

History

The duration of the symptoms, frequency, urgency, nocturia, as well as haematuria need to be established. The patient's age, occupation, presence of chest conditions, constipation, drug history (eg diuretics) as well as drinking (alcohol, beverages) and smoking habits should be recorded. The effect of urinary incontinence on her social life should be assessed, and any associated bowel incontinence, previous incontinence surgery, sexual activity and associated gynaecological problems noted. A past obstetric history is also informative.

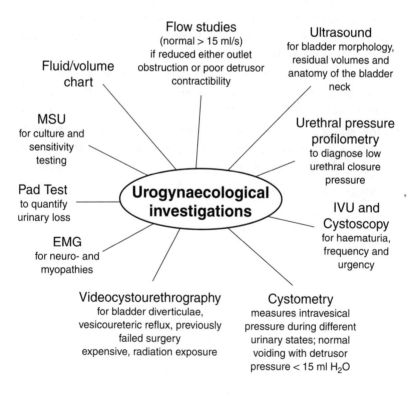

Flow studies
(normal > 15 ml/s)
if reduced either outlet
obstruction or poor detrusor
contractibility

Ultrasound
for bladder morphology,
residual volumes and
anatomy of the bladder
neck

Fluid/volume
chart

MSU
for culture and
sensitivity
testing

Urethral pressure
profilometry
to diagnose low
urethral closure
pressure

Pad Test
to quantify
urinary loss

Urogynaecological investigations

EMG
for neuro- and
myopathies

IVU and
Cystoscopy
for haematuria,
frequency and
urgency

Videocystourethrography
for bladder diverticulae,
vesicoureteric reflux, previously
failed surgery
expensive, radiation exposure

Cystometry
measures intravesical
pressure during different
urinary states; normal
voiding with detrusor
pressure < 15 ml H_2O

Examination

A full general and gynaecological examination should be performed, paying particular attention to chest auscultation, the heart and palpation of the abdomen for the presence of masses. Speculum examination may reveal genital atrophy. A pool of urine might be visible in the case of a fistula, and a co-existent cystocele or rectocele can be detected with a Sim's speculum examination. The pelvic examination focuses on the mobility of the anterior vaginal wall and the presence of pelvic masses like fibroids or ovarian tumours.

A patient with classical frequency, urgency and dysuria should provide a mid-stream urine sample for culture and sensitivity testing. Any infection should be treated, and certainly before embarking on invasive urodynamic studies. In women with mild symptoms a pad test can provide a qualitative assessment of the amount of urinary loss. A fluid/volume chart is cheap, simple, informative and may clarify the patient's drinking habits, eg tea, coffee and should form a baseline investigation. Modification of drinking habits may resolve her symptoms.

If haematuria is present a thorough investigation with cystoscopy and an intravenous urogram to rule out malignancy and other serious pathology is mandatory. Urodynamics is the standard investigation. Its results determine the treatment option employed, for example medical therapy for detrusor instability, pelvic floor exercises and surgical procedure for genuine stress incontinence. Detrusor overactivity might be better detected by ambulatory urodynamics and additional tests such as ultrasound scan for bladder-wall thickness. Videocystourethrography is particularly helpful in patients with previous failed surgery or vesicoureteric reflux. Flow studies might be performed prior to planned surgery since a low flow rate reduces surgical success. An EMG should be done for patients with suspected neuropathy and/or myopathy. Urethral pressure profilometry may detect urethral instability, whilst a simple cystometry can generally differentiate stress from urge incontinence types. CT scanning or MRI are useful in further characterising pelvic masses. If a fistula is suspected, a three-swab test can be performed as well as special radiological investigations such as urethrocystography.

Essay 6

Surgical treatment of vulval carcinoma may cause significant postoperative morbidity.

Describe measures that can be taken to avoid this.

Essay tips
The key words in this question are:

* surgical treatment
* vulval carcinoma
* postoperative morbidity
* describe measures.

Surgical treatment
In dealing with questions on surgery/surgical treatment, it is advisable to plan your answer along the following lines: preoperative, intraoperative and postoperative and follow-up as applicable. The two main parties involved are the patient and the surgeon. The table below illustrates this approach.

	Patient	Surgeon
Preoperative		
Intraoperative		
Postoperative		
Follow-up		

There are constant and recurring themes for the surgeon and for all procedures.

Preoperative
Counselling the patient, explaining the intended benefits of the procedure, the potential complications, failure rates and answering her questions all help to avoid unrealistic expectations and legal claims. A thorough knowledge of her disease and any incidental relevant medical, surgical and gynaecological history. These factors may limit the extent of the procedure(s) undertaken. Involvement of other specialists such as physicians and anaesthetists may be required and should be utilised.

Intraoperative

A good surgical training, in-depth anatomical knowledge, technical expertise and the avoidance of unduly prolonged procedure are essential ingredients in reducing operative morbidity. Other strategies include appropriate incisions, meticulous haemostasis with wound drains as required, antibiotic prophylaxis and thromboprophylaxis.

Postoperative

Regular reviews of the patient on ward rounds with explanations of the procedure and their progress towards recovery help to allay patients' fears. The early recognition of complications is essential, which is facilitated by good communication with nurses, physiotherapists and dieticians to mention but a few.

Other points

These might be the timely uptake of diagnostic facilities (eg chest X-ray) and a properly arranged follow-up.

Vulval carcinoma

The Royal College advocates the regional centralisation of cancer services and referral of patients to these centres within four weeks of diagnosis. This is primarily intended to provide a multidisciplinary team/expert care to achieve optimal outcomes, and secondly, to avoid significant disease progression.

Now consider the patient. She might be old, with a significant medical history and on a multiple-drug regimen. Coexistent gynaecological disease, such as a prolapse, might be present and contribute to postoperative morbidity if a repair is not undertaken simultaneously. So history, examination and appropriate preoperative investigations are important. Since this patient has cancer, the oncology nurse specialist and counsellor should be involved at an early stage, as well as the patient's family (if the patient agrees) and the primary care team. These steps may reduce her psychological morbidity and sense of isolation.

Postoperative morbidity

Bleeding, infection and venous thromboembolism are associated with surgery and these complications need to be addressed in your answer. With respect to surgery for vulval cancer, the reader may find the following diagram helpful.

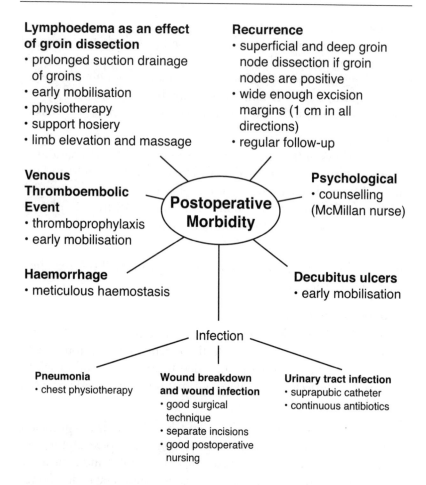

Lymphoedema as an effect of groin dissection
- prolonged suction drainage of groins
- early mobilisation
- physiotherapy
- support hosiery
- limb elevation and massage

Recurrence
- superficial and deep groin node dissection if groin nodes are positive
- wide enough excision margins (1 cm in all directions)
- regular follow-up

Venous Thromboembolic Event
- thromboprophylaxis
- early mobilisation

Postoperative Morbidity

Psychological
- counselling (McMillan nurse)

Haemorrhage
- meticulous haemostasis

Decubitus ulcers
- early mobilisation

Infection

Pneumonia
- chest physiotherapy

Wound breakdown and wound infection
- good surgical technique
- separate incisions
- good postoperative nursing

Urinary tract infection
- suprapubic catheter
- continuous antibiotics

Describe measures

This means describing what can be done. Avoid stating that one 'must'! Use 'might', 'may' and 'could'. The question can be answered satisfactorily by applying common sense. Unfortunately, there are no results from randomised controlled trials upon which to make recommendations for all these factors, so avoid strong language. Examiners don't enjoy receiving orders from candidates!

The essay itself

Detailed attention to pre-, intra- and postoperative care may reduce the burden of postoperative morbidity from vulvectomy. Referral within two weeks to a cancer centre not only allows input from an expert multidisciplinary team, but also reduces significant disease progression.

Preoperatively

Early contact with the oncology counselling nurse and good communication with the patient, her family (if she agrees) and the primary health team may help to reduce psychological morbidity. In addition, early involvement of other specialists, such as physicians and anaesthetists, should be considered

History
A thorough history should be obtained, including her age and details of any medical and drug history.

Examination
A full general and local examination should be performed to assess the extent of her local disease, to carefully plan the optimal surgical procedure and to assess any coexisting gynaecological disease, eg a prolapse. Input from other specialists may be required.

Investigation
Basic investigations and full pre-operative work up should include a full blood count, blood for Group and save U&E; a chest X-ray. Intravenous urogram and ECG may also be required.

Intraoperative

Here, a good surgical technique, an in-depth anatomical knowledge and a sterile technique are important. Proper positioning of the patient, thromboprophylaxis and antibiotics as well as meticulous haemostasis and drains will facilitate the patient's recovery. Simple vulvectomy with lymphadenectomy achieves similar results as radical vulvectomy and lymphadenectomy. The former procedure is, however, associated with much less postoperative wound complications, anatomical distortion and lymphoedema. Therefore, a wide local incision instead of a V (butterfly) incision is preferable. If superficial groin lymph nodes are found to be positive on frozen section histology, then the deep groin nodes should also be removed, since cancer recurrence in the groins is very difficult to treat. Early-stage vulval cancer may be managed with a wide local excision and unilateral groin node dissection: no groin dissection is necessary in stage Ia. Bilateral groin node dissection over separate incisions is, however, needed in patients with central vulval cancer.

Postoperative

Early mobilisation and physiotherapy may help to prevent thromboembolism, decubitus ulcers and pneumonia. Limb elevation and massage, in addition to prolonged suction drainage, may help to reduce the risk of lymphoedema secondary to groin dissection. Good nursing care and judicious antibiotic therapy may help to prevent wound breakdown and infections. Examinations of the patient and reviews of her management will permit early detection of complications.

Follow-up

Regular follow-ups are important so that early treatment can be instituted for recurrences.

Essay 7

Outline the benefits of the levonorgestrel intrauterine system (Mirena coil).

Essay tips
The key words in this question are:

- outline
- benefits
- Mirena coil.

Outline
This sort of question tests your factual knowledge. No in-depth explanations and justifications are needed. Be comprehensive; a clever use of punctuation marks may help if you are short of time. In questions of this nature, no marks are awarded for detailed discussions, irrespective of how persuasive they may be. The question is a straightforward outline and should be treated as such.

Benefits
Mean benefits only. This is no time to discuss the acceptability, difficulties in fitting the coil or subsequent complications. No marks will be awarded for such digressions.

Mirena coil
The figure on the next page outlines some of the important benefits of the Mirena coil.

The essay itself

The Mirena coil is a relatively newly developed intrauterine contraceptive device impregnated with the progestogen levonorgestrel. It is highly effective and fertility quickly returns to normal once it is removed. It has the proven and added benefit of improving menstrual disorders. Mirena has gained wide acceptance for the treatment of menorrhagia and dysmenorrhoea may also improve. There are reports of significant reductions in the number of hysterectomies for benign indications, thereby leading to cost savings for the NHS.

The slow-release levonorgestrel acts locally at the endometrium and effectively treats endometrial hyperplasia. This local delivery avoids the progestogenic side-effects associated with systemic administration during combined hormone-replacement therapy (HRT), and in other circumstances where endometrial protection from estrogen administration is indicated.

The Mirena coil is suggested to relieve symptoms associated with the premenstrual syndrome, probably because of the improvement in menorrhagia and dysmenorrhoea. The use of 17β-estradiol

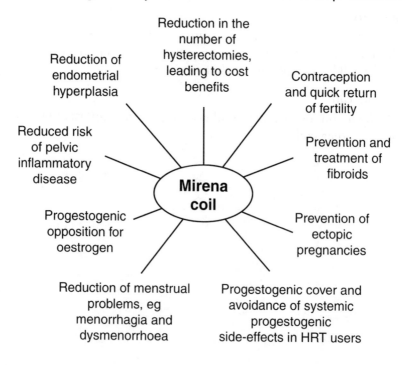

combined with cyclical progestogen is effective in the treatment of premenstrual syndrome. Replacing the progestogenic component with the Mirena coil avoids the exacerbation of premenstrual symptoms attributable to systemic progestogenic side-effects, including headaches, bloating and sore, tender breasts.

Other benefits include the prevention and treatment of fibroids and the prevention of ectopic pregnancies and pelvic inflammatory disease (PID).

Essay 8

Compare and contrast the treatment options for symptomatic endometriosis.

Essay tips

The key words in this question are:

- compare
- contrast
- treatment options
- symptomatic
- endometriosis.

Compare

This means highlighting the similarities. What do these treatment options have in common?

Contrast

What are the differences between them?

Example: The hormonal treatments all interfere with conception. However, gonadotrophin-releasing hormone (GnRH) analogues are better tolerated than danazol. The oral contraceptive pill has a similar effect as GnRH analogues in terms of symptom relief, but is a cheaper option.

Treatment options

Symptomatic endometriosis is treated conservatively, surgically or with alternative therapies. Conservative treatment can be divided into hormonal and non-hormonal treatment. Surgical treatment may also be divided into conservative (to retain fertility) or radical, laparoscopic or open surgery. Alternative therapies include acupuncture and hypnosis.

Symptomatic

The symptoms of endometriosis include dysmenorrhoea, deep dyspareunia, pelvic pain and subfertility. Furthermore, the symptoms may be mild, moderate or severe, and may have an adverse effect on the woman's personal and/or professional life.

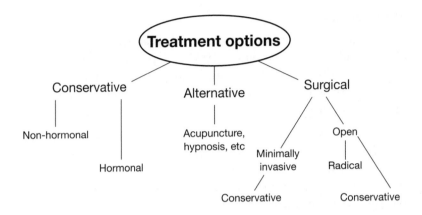

Endometriosis

Remember that endometriosis may affect women at any stage of their reproductive life, say from 15 to 45 years of age. The women may be parous or nulligravid and subfertile. Some may have coexistent gynaecological problems. Don't approach this question with streamlined statements such as 'a 22-year-old with pelvic pain and mild endometriosis – Panadol'. That's not even a fraction of the story.

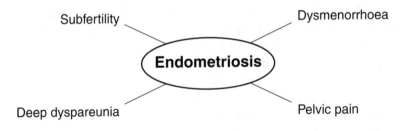

The essay itself

Endometriosis is a common disease with a poorly understood aetiology. It affects approximately 10% of reproductive-age women. Treatment options may be medical, surgical or alternative and are generally considered in context with the patient's history, findings on physical/pelvic examination and other investigations.

The symptoms of endometriosis and their severity correlate very poorly with laparoscopic findings and the American Fertility Society scoring system. The main symptoms are dysmenorrhoea, pelvic pain, dyspareunia and infertility – less commonly rectal bleeding, haematuria and urgency.

Conservative treatment

Non-hormonal

Non-hormonal medical treatments include the prostaglandin synthetase inhibitors (eg mefenamic acid). These are effective in relieving dysmenorrhoea and pelvic pain, and have the advantage that fertility is not impaired.

Hormonal

Hormonal treatments are effective in providing symptom relief but they all interfere with fertility. Moreover, there is a significant chance of recurrence of endometriosis once treatment is discontinued. The oral contraceptive pill relieves dysmenorrhoea and dyspareunia and may be a suitable option for young women with mild symptoms who do not wish to become pregnant. Progestogens achieve symptom relief in 80% of cases, but there is some concern about increasing the risk for cardiovascular disease in the long term. Danazol may be given for three months (200–600 mg/day), but is not well tolerated because of its androgenic side-effects. Gestrinone given orally twice-weekly is as effective as danazol but has a better side-effect profile. GnRH analogues are particularly effective in women with superficial lesions and relieve symptoms in 90% of women. However, it is expensive, the injection is uncomfortable, it is ineffective against endometriomas of more than 3 cm and may be associated with marked vasomotor symptoms. They also have adverse effects on bone density. 'Add-back' hormone therapy may reduce vasomotor symptoms and prevent bone loss, allowing more prolonged use of GnRH analogues, ie beyond the usual six months. Mifepristone (RU486), tamoxifen and gosopyl need further clinical evaluation.

Surgical treatment

Surgery aims to restore pelvic anatomy in fertile women or to interrupt the sensory pathways in symptomatic patients, it may be performed laparoscopically or as an open procedure. The cure would be total abdominal hysterectomy and bilateral salpingo-oophorectomy: this may be offered to women who have completed their families and/or who have coexistent gynaecological disease such as large fibroids and menorrhagia. All surgical options carry the potential risk of bleeding, infection and venous thromboembolism, and, particularly in endometriosis, damage to the bowel, ureter and bladder. Laparoscopic laser vaporisation or coagulation of endometriotic deposits improves fertility, while nerve ablation of the uterosacral ligaments achieves a 60% improvement in symptoms.

Alternative therapies

Alternative methods, such as acupuncture or hypnotherapy, may work in motivated subjects and no side-effects are known. However, their effectiveness is yet to be proven in randomised trials.

Essay 9

Review the effects of medical treatment for the relief of menopausal symptoms.

Essay tips

The key words in this question are:

- review
- effects
- medical treatment
- menopausal symptoms.

Review

To date the RCOG has yet to use the word 'review' in its essay questions, but it may come up at some stage.

'Review' is the broadest possible approach to an essay, and, ideally, the candidate should summarise the facts into subheadings and then discuss these as one topic. For example, when answering a 'review' question:

- Instead of writing 'The Marshall–Marchetti–Krantz operation, Burch colposuspension and Aldridge sling are used for the surgical treatment of genuine stress incontinence', you could choose to discuss these procedures under the subheading 'Suprapubic procedures used for genuine stress incontinence', then discuss them together giving one or two examples.
- Instead of writing 'Amniocentesis, chorionic villus sampling and fetal blood sampling can be used to determine the fetal karyotype', consider discussing them under the subheading 'Invasive prenatal diagnostic tests'.
- Instead of writing 'Changes in liver function tests, urea and electrolytes and uric acid assist in the diagnosis of pre-eclampsia', consider summarising these changes under the subheading 'Changes in blood biochemistry'.

Begin by 'brainstorming' the raw facts, think of suitable subheadings, and then organise the essay around these. This will save time and paper and will give you the opportunity to cover the spectrum of the question.

Effects

Effects include potential benefits and harmful effects. Under the suggested subheadings given above, you could say:

- 'Suprapubic procedures used for the surgical treatment of genuine stress incontinence (GSI), achieve a cure rate of 80–90% over 5 years. However, all these procedures have the morbidity problems of major surgery, eg blood loss, scars, etc.'
- 'Invasive prenatal diagnostic tests reliably determine the fetal karyotype, but are all associated with a risk of fetal loss.'
- 'Blood biochemistry assists in the diagnosis of pre-eclampsia, but all parameters need to be appraised in context with other clinical and haematological findings.'

Medical treatment

Note that this is not an HRT question! It neither asks for the different routes of delivering hormone replacement therapy, nor does it deal with the question of who should take HRT and who shouldn't. The medical treatment options are:

- estrogen
- progestogens
- tibolone
- phytoestrogens
- clonidine
- testosterone
- antidepressants.

Menopausal symptoms

Subheadings are required here – eg hot flushes and night sweats should be discussed under 'Vasomotor symptoms'; vaginal dryness and sexual satisfaction under 'Urogenital symptoms'; and so on.

These categories now need to be appraised in context with medical treatment. Each of the medical treatment subheadings may then deal with vasomotor symptoms, the urogenital system, etc, separately – preferably divided into paragraphs.

The essay itself

Over 80% of women experience at least one menopausal symptom. Medical treatment aims to prevent and/or treat these symptoms and improve quality of life with minimal adverse effects.

Estrogens

Estrogens are proven to relieve vasomotor symptoms and improve urogenital symptoms and depressed moods. There is also some evidence that estrogens might prevent, or at least slow, the onset of Alzheimer's disease. Randomised controlled trials have shown that treatment improves quality of life and wellbeing.

However, estrogen therapy is associated with the short-term side-effects of weight gain and breast tenderness. Long-term adverse effects include: an increased risk of venous thromboembolism, endometrial cancer and breast cancer – the latter returning to the background risk five or more years after stopping treatment.

Progestogens

In randomised trials, progestogens have been shown to reduce vasomotor symptoms. However, they exert no beneficial effects on bone density.

Progestogens are associated with various side-effects, including: breast tenderness, bloating, water retention and mood changes.

Tibolone

Tibolone significantly improves vasomotor symptoms, libido and vaginal lubrication. Sexual satisfaction is reported to be better with tibolone than with sequential hormone replacement therapy. Bone density increases, but the reports of effects on psychological symptoms and quality of life are conflicting.

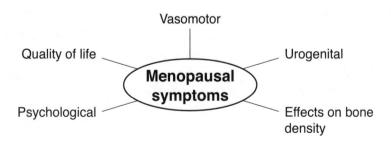

The chief unwanted effect associated with the use of tibolone is breakthrough bleeding, which occurs in approximately 10% of users.

Phytoestrogens

Phytoestrogens, which may be found in soy flour, relieve the frequency and severity of vasomotor symptoms. Their effects on urogenital atrophy, psychological wellbeing and quality of life await further research.

There are no known harmful effects.

Clonidine

Clonidine reduces vasomotor symptoms and has no more unwanted effects than placebo.

Testosterone

Testosterone improves sexual enjoyment and libido. Although reduced doses of estrogen may be needed to control vasomotor symptoms, its effects on psychological symptoms and quality of life are undergoing further studies.

There is no increase in the incidence of adverse androgenic effects when testosterone is used in approved replacement doses of 50–100 mg every six months.

Antidepressants

Antidepressants and their effects on menopausal symptoms have not been thoroughly studied. However, there are well-documented harmful side-effects associated with this class of drugs, including: sedation and agitation; urinary and visual problems; liver dysfunction; and cardiac dysrhythmias.

Essay 10

Laparoscopic-assisted vaginal hysterectomy should be the preferred method for removal of the uterus.

Debate this statement.

Essay tips

The key words in this question are:
- laparoscopic-assisted vaginal hysterectomy
- should be the preferred method
- removal of the uterus
- debate.

Laparoscopic-assisted vaginal hysterectomy (LAVH)

As a surgical procedure, the usual considerations listed below will apply.

- cost of equipment
- duration of procedure
- blood loss
- analgesia requirements
- recovery time/return to normal
- surgical training
- patient selection, eg obesity, previous abdominal surgery
- cosmetic results.

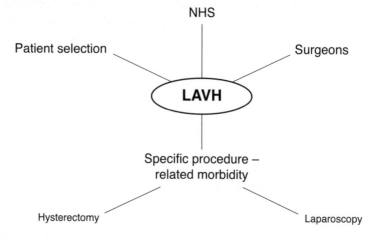

The candidate should avoid an open-ended, unstructured answer because of the word 'debate'. In this exam there is limited room for non evidence-based personal opinions. Therefore, develop a plan and stick to it!

Should be the preferred method

What procedure is laparoscopic-assisted vaginal hysterectomy (LAVH) competing with? – Total abdominal hysterectomy (TAH) and vaginal hysterectomy (VH). Do not spend the entire essay on laparoscopic-assisted vaginal hysterectomy! Revisit the essay plan and replace LAVH with TAH and comment on the four main aspects (NHS, surgeons, patient selection and specific procedure-related morbidity), and finally do the same for vaginal hysterectomy. Then, and only then, can you judge whether LAVH should be the preferred method or not.

Examples

- Although the operation time is longer with LAVH compared to TAH or VH, there is as little blood loss as with VH.

- Patients' analgesia requirements, recovery time and length of hospital stay are far less than for TAH.

- The equipment for laparoscopic hysterectomy is certainly expensive, but the method still appears to be cost-effective for the reasons mentioned above.

- If associated gynaecological problems were suspected, eg endometriosis, LAVH would be the preferred method over VH, since the diagnosis and treatment can be offered at the same time.

Removal of the uterus

This indicates that conservative procedures/interventions should be left out. Clearly, there is no room for a discussion or debate on the Mirena coil.

Debate

'Debate' implies that the examiner is not expecting a 'yes' or 'no' response. Debate invites a comparison of LAVH versus TAH versus VH. In other words, in what areas is LAVH superior to TAH and VH or under what circumstances would a TAH still be indicated or a vaginal hysterectomy preferred?

The essay itself

Laparoscopic-assisted vaginal hysterectomy (LAVH) aims to convert a total abdominal hysterectomy (TAH) into a vaginal procedure, or to complete a difficult vaginal hysterectomy (VH) instead of converting it into an abdominal one. By definition, the uterine arteries are divided laparoscopically.

On the one hand, LAVH enjoys all the advantages of minimally invasive surgery, including good cosmetic results, reduced postoperative analgesia requirements, shorter hospital stay and a quicker return of patients to their normal activities. With respect to these, it competes favourably with vaginal hysterectomy and, despite the prolonged operation time and cost of equipment, it is still cost-effective. The average blood loss is also less than with TAH.

However, training of surgeons and acquisition of the necessary skills takes longer than for TAH or VH.

If associated gynaecological problems were suspected (eg endometriosis), laparoscopic-assisted vaginal hysterectomy would be the preferred method over vaginal hysterectomy, since both diagnosis and treatment can be offered at the same operation. Nevertheless, TAH is still the operation of choice for patients with large tumours, since the operation offers good access, visualisation and tactile information of the whole pelvis and the abdomen as well as the opportunity for omentectomy, lymphadenectomy and easier adnexectomy. Obese patients with previous abdominal surgery and adhesions are more at risk of complications at laparoscopy (eg damage to blood vessels and bowel), and therefore need careful assessment. Difficulties with VH arise when there is poor access, an enlarged immobile uterus and/or suspected adnexal pathology. Laparoscopy is the 'gold standard' investigation of adnexal/pelvic pathology and has replaced laparotomy and TAH for this indication. It combines the ability of diagnosis with treatment, eg for endometriosis.

In summary, LAVH may be of benefit for some patients who would otherwise have had a TAH, but LAVH has little to add in cases where a VH is possible.

Essay 11

Ovarian hyperstimulation syndrome (OHSS) is a potentially severe complication of supraphysiological ovarian stimulation.

Outline the measures that can be taken to prevent OHSS.

Essay tips
The key words in this question are:

- all of the first sentence
- outline
- measures
- to prevent OHSS.

All of the first sentence
The candidate is not asked to discuss or debate this statement. So, it should just be noted and treated as it is. Do not use it as an introduction in your essay either; such a move lacks originality.

Outline
Confine yourself to factual information without giving explanations, and use short and concise sentences. If you're in a hurry, commas between facts will suffice.

Measures
Patients' selection is important. Who would be at an increased risk of OHSS?

Well, women who:

- are young
- are slim
- have polycystic ovaries
- have a previous history of OHSS.

In questions dealing with risk factors, morbidity and complications (eg in surgery), the candidate should consider the principle of 'patient selection'. It gives the examiner the impression that 'you know what you are doing'. You might earn some marks even if you forgot some details. The other aspect of the measures to reduce OHSS, deals with the interventions, for example variation of drugs, monitoring hormone levels or cancellation of cycles.

Another major consideration relates to who should be undertaking the procedure and where it should be done. Referral to specialists for treatment in dedicated units is an important step in reducing the risk of OHSS.

An essay plan for such a question might look like this:

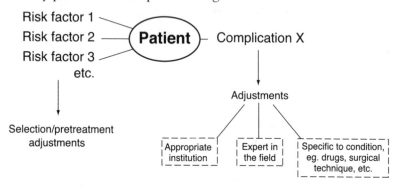

To prevent OHSS

The recognition that OHSS is closely related to the use of gonadotrophins prior to assisted conception is the key to a good answer. This complication is only very rarely associated with the use of anti-estrogens.

Non-pharmacological preventive measures include:
- diet for obese women with polycystic ovarian syndrome (PCOS)
- laparoscopic ovarian drill for women with PCOS who are clomifene-resistant
- ultrasound scan monitoring of ovarian response
- cancellation of cycles with an excessive ovarian response
- monitoring of serum estradiol levels
- cryopreservation of all embryos.

Pharmacological measures can be:
- replacement of the gonadotrophin-releasing hormone (GnRH) analogues/human menopausal gonadotrophin (HMG) regime with purified follicle-stimulating hormone (FSH) using the low-dose incremental regime

- withholding of the ovulatory human chorionic gonadotrophin (HCG) injection in cycles with excessive ovarian response
- discontinuation of gonadotrophin administration and delayed HCG injection in cycles with high serum estradiol levels
- use of recombinant luteinising hormone (LH) instead of HCG for final follicular maturation
- replacement of HCG by progesterone for luteal-phase support
- intravenous albumin administration at the time of oocyte retrieval
- immunomodulation may be used in the future.

The essay itself

The prevention of ovarian hyperstimulation syndrome (OHSS) starts with the selection of patients and recognition of their risk factors. Special attention should be paid to young and thin women, women with polycystic ovaries and women with a previous history of OHSS as these groups are at increased risk.

Referral to an expert in assisted conception in a dedicated in-vitro fertilisation (IVF) unit would be the first step.

Non-pharmacological preventive measures include: a diet programme for obese patients with polycystic ovarian syndrome (PCOS) and laparoscopic ovarian drill for women with clomifene-resistant PCOS.

Ultrasound scans may be used to monitor ovarian response, and cancellation should be considered for cycles with excessive ovarian response, although this may trigger some degree of psychological morbidity in the affected couple. Measurement of serum estradiol levels is also important in high-risk women as well as cryopreservation of all embryos.

It is well documented that OHSS is closely related to the use of gonadotrophins prior to assisted conception. On the other hand, anti-estrogens are only rarely associated with severe OHSS. Therefore, the cautious use of gonadotrophins and manipulation of treatment within the pharmacological group may help to reduce severe OHSS. Purified FSH given by the low-dose incremental regime can replace the GnRH analogue/HMG regime. In cycles with excessive ovarian response the ovulatory HCG can be withheld. Also in cycles with high serum estradiol levels, discontinuation of gonadotrophin administration and delayed HCG injection is effective in reducing the risk of OHSS. Recombinant LH instead of HCG should be used for final follicular maturation. Progesterone has been shown to be as effective as HCG for luteal-phase support and could be a safer option. Albumin can be given intravenously at the time of oocyte retrieval to enhance oncotic pressure and reduce the risk of OHSS.

Studies on immunomodulation are currently in progress and this approach may be used in the future to prevent severe OHSS in high-risk patients.

Essay 12

You are called to theatre by your SHO who was about to perform a termination of pregnancy (TOP) at 12 weeks' gestation but reports that he has perforated the uterus. You are the most senior doctor available.

How would you deal with this situation?

Essay tips

The key words in this question are:

- the scenario as described in the first two sentences
- how would you deal with this situation.

The scenario as described in the first two sentences

Imagine you've just received this phone call. You make your way to the theatre. What are your thoughts? (Not – 'Oh my God, why me?')

Communication

Discuss your own plan with the theatre sister and the anaesthetist. You plan to do a laparoscopy in the first instance but may proceed to laparotomy. Let them make arrangements, eg set up for a laparotomy, call a consultant anaesthetist and inform a general surgeon if necessary. Since there is a medicolegal aspect to this case, think of:

- good clinical notes
- giving a clear explanation to the patient, your consultant, the patient's GP and the risk manager later on.

To obtain good marks in this essay, mention the medicolegal aspects and the adjustments you would make.

Monitoring

Blood loss, haemoglobin levels, clotting results, oxygen saturations, urinary output, etc all need to be monitored by the anaesthetist.

A full blood count, crossmatch of at least two units of blood.

Treatment

Obviously the aim is to evacuate the uterus, to achieve haemostasis and to ensure that neighbouring structures such as the bladder and bowel are intact. Now think of different scenarios, eg:

- small hole, not actively bleeding → expectant management with antibiotics and oxytocics
- moderately sized tear, moderate blood loss → laparotomy and haemostatic sutures, inspection of bladder and bowel
- large tear with massive bleeding → laparotomy, attempt at homeostatic suture, if not succeeding proceed to hysterectomy, involvement of the bowel surgeon to rule out bowel injuries, etc.

How would you deal with this situation?

It is essentially a management question. As for any other management question it may be structured into history, examination, investigation, treatment and follow-up.

History

You want to check the gestation, whether it is a bicornuate uterus, how much blood has been lost so far and what was the perforating instrument.

Examination

Another quick look through the speculum gives some idea of the blood loss and a pelvic examination will give an estimate of the size of the uterus.

Investigation

An ultrasound-guided evacuation of the uterus could be helpful in addition to the diagnostic laparoscopy.

Treatment

This has already been discussed.

Follow-up

It is vitally important to see this patient in the out-patients clinic. First of all to ensure that she has fully recovered and, secondly, to clarify the matter of contraception.

Essay plan
Your essay plan could work like this:

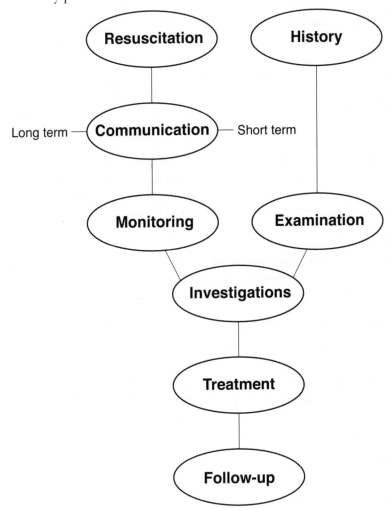

The essay itself

A perforated, pregnant uterus represents an emergency situation.

Emergency action

Resuscitation starts with the placement of another intravenous line and appropriate fluid replacement. If the patient is not intubated the anaesthetist should consider this and the patient be ventilated artificially. The theatre sister should make the appropriate arrangements, for a laparascopy and a laparotomy, call a consultant anaesthetist if required and inform the general surgeon if necessary.

History

A quick history will clarify the gestational age of the pregnancy, whether to expect a bicornuate uterus, how much blood was lost so far, and what instrument perforated the uterus.

Examination

A speculum examination will give some information about the blood loss and a bimanual examination should be performed to assess the size of the uterus.

Investigations

The anaesthetist should obtain blood samples for a full blood count and for crossmatching of at least two units. A diagnostic laparoscopy should be done swiftly. Safe evacuation of the uterus may be best achieved under ultrasound guidance. Haemoglobin levels, clotting results, oxygen saturations and urinary output need to be monitored and, of course, the blood loss.

Treatment

Treatment, first of all, aims to evacuate the uterus, and also to assess the size and location of the perforation and to achieve haemostasis. At the same time assurance is needed that neighbouring structures such as the bladder and bowel are intact. Therefore a diagnostic laparoscopy in the first instance is mandatory. A small perforation not actively bleeding may be managed expectantly, covering the patient with antibiotics and giving her oxytocics. An average-sized tear in the uterus bleeding moderately may be controlled by pressure. Failing that a laparotomy is required. Haemostatic sutures can be applied, and the bladder and bowel inspected for possible damage. If in any doubt, a general surgeon should be called to help. A large perforation bleeding massively may necessitate a hysterectomy for haemostatic purposes, and to ensure the patient's survival. This decision should not be postponed unnecessarily but taken by senior members of the multidisciplinary team. Arrangements may need to be made to transfer the patient postoperatively to a high-dependency unit and thromboprophylaxis should be prescribed.

Follow-up

Since there is a medicolegal aspect to this scenario, the risk manager, the consultant and the patient's GP should be informed as soon as possible. A clear explanation should be given to the patient and good and legible operative notes kept. Follow-up arrangements should be made regardless of the severity of the perforation to ensure the patient has recovered fully and also to discuss contraception. For medicolegal purposes it would be important to see this patient in the future to clarify any questions she or her partner may have and to give her all the support she needs.

Essay 13

Discuss the impact of diagnostic radiology on the management of gynaecological patients.

Essay tips

The key words in this question are:

- discuss
- diagnostic radiology
- management
- gynaecological patients.

Discuss

The College expects you to give an appraisal of the impact of radiology in our field. Obviously, there are many advantages to having a few machines available. However, the specific benefits and drawbacks need to be highlighted. Topics such as radiation exposure, pain during radiological investigations, the reliability of results and their limitations and expense should be discussed.

Diagnostic radiology

Not radiotherapy! 'What sort of radiological investigations can be performed for gynaecological patients?' 'What kind of machines are available?' There is no reason to panic because you do know the answer. Yes, simple X-rays, X-rays with contrast, CT scanning, MRI and radionuclide imaging can all be performed. You can now construct an essay plan.

Example opposite.

Management

Whatever radiology has to offer is, and will be, an investigation result. It is an example of an essay where history, examination, etc do not apply. As suggested in the essay plan, the question is which patient with what problem would benefit from what kind of diagnostic radiological investigation? And, indeed, how much influence has the result on the treatment of the patient?

A symptomatic patient with a perfusion defect on a V/Q scan is very likely to have a pulmonary embolism and so will be

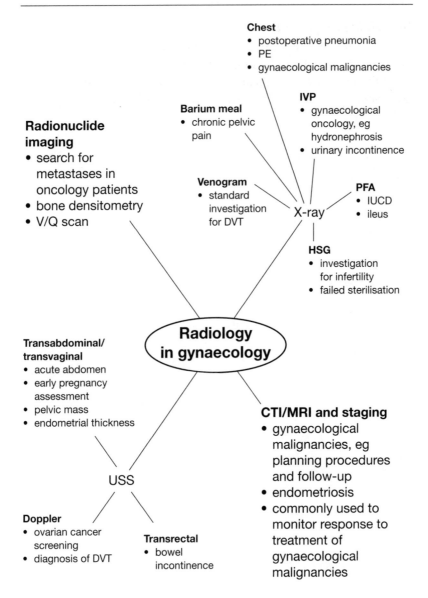

Chest
- postoperative pneumonia
- PE
- gynaecological malignancies

IVP
- gynaecological oncology, eg hydronephrosis
- urinary incontinence

Barium meal
- chronic pelvic pain

Radionuclide imaging
- search for metastases in oncology patients
- bone densitometry
- V/Q scan

Venogram
- standard investigation for DVT

PFA
- IUCD
- ileus

X-ray

HSG
- investigation for infertility
- failed sterilisation

Radiology in gynaecology

Transabdominal/ transvaginal
- acute abdomen
- early pregnancy assessment
- pelvic mass
- endometrial thickness

USS

Doppler
- ovarian cancer screening
- diagnosis of DVT

Transrectal
- bowel incontinence

CTI/MRI and staging
- gynaecological malignancies, eg planning procedures and follow-up
- endometriosis
- commonly used to monitor response to treatment of gynaecological malignancies

heparinised. However, a postmenopausal woman with an endometrial thickness of 6 mm on ultrasound scan has a very small chance of endometrial cancer. She needs more investigations, namely a hysteroscopy and endometrial biopsy.

Gynaecological patients

They do not all have cancer! The field of gynaecology includes oncology, gynaecological endocrinology, infertility and urogynaecology. Of course, early pregnancy management is included as well; an area where patients might enjoy having a radiological investigation.

The essay itself

Rapid progress has been made in the field of diagnostic radiology over the past few decades, and it is now a cornerstone of gynaecological practice.

Ultrasound scan, either abdominal or transvaginal, assists in the diagnosis of early pregnancy, polycystic ovarian syndrome and ovarian cysts (for which Doppler might be added). Although it forms part of the screening process for ovarian cancer, more research is in progress to improve its sensitivity and specificity. Fibroids can be visualised and endometrial thickness measured in women with postmenopausal bleeding. It generally assists in the diagnosis of uterine and adnexal pathology. A transrectal ultrasound scan is used in post partum patients with faecal or flatus incontinence to assess competence of the anal sphincter. Doppler ultrasound has more recently been endorsed in the diagnosis of deep vein thrombosis. However, a venogram is still the 'gold standard', despite being painful, exposing the patient to radiation and having the risk of thrombus transport to the lungs. A V/Q scan is performed to diagnose or exclude pulmonary embolism – one of the main complications of gynaecological surgery. Chest X-rays assist in the diagnosis of metastatic gynaecological disease, and also of postoperative pneumonia, pulmonary oedema and embolism. A plain film of the abdomen is used to localise a coil and to diagnose ileus postoperatively. A barium meal might be necessary in the diagnosis of chronic pelvic pain. Intravenous pyelogram is used in the assessment and staging of gynaecological tumours, for example hydronephrosis in cervical cancer, and also in patients with urinary incontinence. Hysterosalpingography is used in the diagnosis of lesions associated with infertility and may help to detect a tubal patency in failed sterilisation.

X-ray investigations are well established but have the disadvantage of radiation exposure, and are potentially carcinogenic. In gynaecological oncology, CT scanning and MRI are mainly used in diagnosis and treatment planning, as well as in the detection of recurrent disease. MRI is rarely used for the diagnosis of endometriosis but can assist in the diagnosis of intoactive endometriotic nodules and in planning management. The advantage of MRI is that it involves no radiation exposure at all; however, it is expensive and not universally available. A copper IUCD would contraindicate an MRI, or it would need to be removed prior to MRI. Caution has to be exercised in patients with epilepsy and those with myocardial infarction. Radionuclide imaging can be used for detecting metastatic disease in bones, and also for measuring bone density. There is, however, some concern about whether these investigations might be carcinogenic.

Obstetrics essays

Essay 14

A 23-year-old primigravid woman has a scan at 30 weeks' gestation, which shows severe intrauterine growth restriction (IUGR).

Discuss your further management.

Essay tips
The key words in this question are:

- 23-year-old woman
- primigravida
- 30 weeks' gestation
- severe IUGR
- management.

23-year-old woman
Age is probably irrelevant in this case. However, whenever age comes up in a question consider pregnancy complications at the extremes of the reproductive years – eg premature births are commoner in teenage and older women; and chromosomal abnormalities of the fetus, multiple pregnancy, pregnancy-induced hypertension, gestational diabetes, placental insufficiency and miscarriage are all commoner in older women.

Primigravida
Induction of labour is more likely to fail in primigravids certainly at such an early gestation, making delivery by Caesarean section more likely; this is particularly the case since severely growth restricted babies may not tolerate labour well.

30 weeks' gestation
'Prematurity', 'steroids', 'neonatologist', 'transfer to tertiary centre' are the associated key words whenever the gestational age is less than 34 weeks.

Severe IUGR
In situations where the baby is considered too big or too small and/or in need of delivery – recheck the dates first. IUGR may be

symmetrical, having an intrinsic cause (eg Down's syndrome), or asymmetrical, whereby placental insufficiency due to an extrinsic cause is more likely (eg pre-eclampsia). Early-onset insults of extrinsic origin may produce symmetrical growth restriction.

Management

Consider the mother and the fetus – a multidisciplinary team approach involving senior obstetricians, paediatricians and anaesthetists as the minimum is almost always applicable. You should also involve the parents in the decision-making process. Management is based on the findings in the history, examination and investigations. In this question the diagnosis has already been made, so these elements of management should be brief and focused on the relevant points. Commonly, and IUGR is a good example, delivery and its potential hazards need to be balanced against close surveillance. The modes of delivery and their associated problems need to be discussed: for example, induction of labour and its potential failure, and Caesarean section and the risk of postpartum haemorrhage (PPH), infection, thromboembolism and a reduced chance of subsequent vaginal delivery. Consider the essay plan on the next page.

By filling in the boxes first you already have your essay structure and, secondly, things might come to mind much quicker. You are less likely to forget the big points like Doppler waveform studies or PET-bloods.

	Maternal	Fetal	Placental
History	Smoking, alcohol, drug abuse Racial background Underlying illness, eg renal disease Pregnancy-associated problems, eg PET, infection	Booking/dating scan Results from FAS Multiple pregnancy	Placenta praevia
Examination	Full general exam, SFH, BP	Presentation	
Investigations	PET-bloods Renal function test TORCH screen Urine for C/S Protein, creatinine clearance and thrombophilia screens	Scan: repeat FAS, if abnormal add amnio, CVS or fetal-blood sampling for karyotype; EFW, presentation, liquor volume, Doppler, BPP, CTG	Scan: localise placenta, single umbilical artery, insertio velamentosa, etc
Treatment	Reduce risk factors, stop smoking, treat underlying medical disorders	Surveillance versus preterm delivery: set criteria, when you would do what; steroids	

Abbreviations: PET, pre-eclamptic toxaemia; FAS, fetal anomaly scan; SFH, stroma-free haemoglobin; BP, blood pressure; TORCH, toxoplasmosis, other infection [congenital syphilis and viruses], rubella, cytomegalovirus, herpes simplex virus; C/S, culture and sensitivity testing; CVS, chorionic villus sampling; EFW, estimated fetal weight; BPP, biophysical profile; CTG, cardiotocography.

The essay itself

IUGR is a condition characterised by failure of the fetus to achieve its full growth potential. It is present in 50–60% of fetuses diagnosed as 'small for gestational age' (SGA), variably defined as less than the third, fifth and tenth centiles for gestational age. The growth restriction may be symmetrical or asymmetrical.

History

Essential points to note in the maternal history include smoking, alcohol and drug use and her racial background. Pre-existing medical disorders may be present, for instance renal or collagen disease and pregnancy-related problems, such as pre-eclampsia. A history of infection and antiphospholipid antibody should be explored.

The 'fetal history' starts by checking dates and the results of a triple test and fetal anomaly scan. Multiple pregnancy should be excluded.

Examination

A full general and obstetric examination should be performed, noting the symphyseal fundal height, maternal blood pressure, urinalysis and fetal presentation.

Investigations

Maternal investigations should include a full blood count, U&E, liver function tests, uric acid and coagulation screen if the blood pressure is elevated, and a TORCH screen may be added and urine sent for culture and sensitivity testing. A 24-hour urine collection made for protein and creatinine clearance measurements if there is proteinuria should be undertaken as these are associated with IVGR.

The main investigation of the fetus is a detailed ultrasound scan determining biparietal diameter (BPD) and abdominal circumference, as well as a repeat fetal anomaly scan. Amniocentesis, or fetal blood sampling may be performed to determine the karyotype if dysmorphic features are suspected. Cordocentesis is especially useful for a TORCH screen. Fetal blood pH can be measured to assess any underlying hypoxia or acidaemia. The fetal weight can be estimated, the presentation checked and the liquor volume determined. Placenta praevia should be ruled out. A biophysical profile may be undertaken and Doppler studies of the umbilical, middle cerebral artery and the ductus venosus carried out to assist in the timing of delivery. A CTG is also useful.

Management

A multidisciplinary approach to management should be adopted, involving obstetricians, neonatologists and anaesthetists. Referral to a tertiary centre may be necessary. The parents should be closely involved in decisions. Admission of the mother and reduction of risk factors (smoking, alcohol and drug abuse, etc) may be required. Steroids in the form of betamethasone should be administered to enhance fetal organ maturation and reduce the risks of respiratory distress syndrome, major intraventricular haemorrhage and necrotising enterocolitis. The balance here is between surveillance, with the attendant risk of intrauterine death, and the delivery of a preterm, compromised fetus. Delivery of a nulliparous woman at 30 weeks' gestation will most probably require a Caesarean section since the cervix is unlikely to respond to induction of labour. Expectant management could be applied in a chromosomally abnormal fetus, a genetically small fetus or where Doppler and CTG assessments are satisfactory. Delivery is indicated in cases of severe oligohydramnios associated with absent or reversed end-diastolic flow or severe intercurrent maternal illness.

Essay 15

Discuss the impact of prepregnancy clinics on future obstetric outcome.

Essay tips

The key words in this question are:

- discuss
- prepregnancy clinics
- obstetric outcome.

Discuss

This question invites you to examine the potential benefits and value of the activities and interventions undertaken in these clinics. Do you think they have made a difference? Do their benefits justify the resources expended? First, what groups of women are candidate attendees to such a clinic? What could be done for women with a previous bad obstetric history, those with medical conditions (eg heart problems), those with a family history of genetic disorders, etc? Their medical notes could be reviewed, treatment for their medical conditions could be optimised and they could be helped to plan a pregnancy so that conception occurred during a relatively disease-free interval. Adjustments of drugs, genetic counselling and tests for potential parents can also be offered. You should present and discuss any published data showing the effect of these strategies on the outcome of subsequent pregnancy.

Prepregnancy clinics

There is ongoing debate whether these clinics justify their costs. Although the body of literature is sparse, the RCOG wants to hear your opinion regardless.

Obstetric outcome

Address the entire perinatal outcome, including the mother, the baby and any potential morbidity or mortality. Prepregnancy clinics are based on the belief that a review and assessment of pre-existing disease to inform decisions on whether a pregnancy is safe or not, early reduction of the impact of disease and counselling would translate to a better perinatal outcome. This approach is supported by data from pregnancies in diabetic patients. However, do not write an essay entirely on genetic counselling and do not forget to mention the partner.

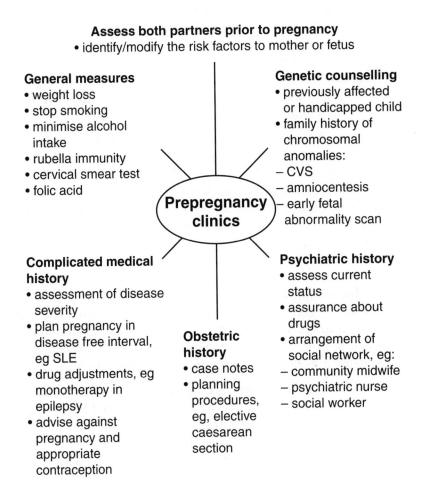

Assess both partners prior to pregnancy
- identify/modify the risk factors to mother or fetus

General measures
- weight loss
- stop smoking
- minimise alcohol intake
- rubella immunity
- cervical smear test
- folic acid

Prepregnancy clinics

Genetic counselling
- previously affected or handicapped child
- family history of chromosomal anomalies:
  - CVS
  - amniocentesis
  - early fetal abnormality scan

Complicated medical history
- assessment of disease severity
- plan pregnancy in disease free interval, eg SLE
- drug adjustments, eg monotherapy in epilepsy
- advise against pregnancy and appropriate contraception

Obstetric history
- case notes
- planning procedures, eg, elective caesarean section

Psychiatric history
- assess current status
- assurance about drugs
- arrangement of social network, eg:
  - community midwife
  - psychiatric nurse
  - social worker

The essay itself

Prepregnancy clinics make the earliest possible attempt to reduce maternal and perinatal morbidity and mortality. Ideally, both partners should be involved. Certain general measures are applicable to all women planning a pregnancy. These include ensuring/advising: optimal body weight; cessation of smoking and recreational drugs/substances, including alcohol; immunity to rubella; up-to-date cervical smear; folic acid supplementation, with the higher dose given to women on anticonvulsant drugs and those with a previous child/children affected by a neural tube defect.

Couples carrying abnormal genetic alleles could receive genetic counselling about the risk of their offspring inheriting the disease. The same applies to couples with a family history of genetic disease or a previous handicapped child. Recurrence risks can be estimated and preimplantation diagnosis offered. Close liaison with the obstetric unit would allow an early booking scan to plan an invasive prenatal diagnostic test, eg chorionic villus sampling or amniocentesis to determine fetal sex (X-linked conditions). This might be preceded by non-invasive tests such as nuchal translucency. The overall objective of these interventions is to prevent or detect the transmission of genetic disorders early and to offer termination of pregnancy if this is the wish of the couple. Such a reduction in the incidence of congenital/chromosomal disorders is expected to translate into a reduction in the perinatal mortality rate.

Women with a medical history could undergo a thorough assessment of their disease status, and a pregnancy planned for conception during a disease-free interval, eg systemic lupus. Drug regimens could be adjusted to reduce/prevent the risk of fetal malformations, eg monotherapy in epileptics. Advice against pregnancy and appropriate contraception might be given: for example, to women with severe cardiac disease to reduce their risk of maternal morbidity and mortality.

Women with cervical insufficiency and recurrent mid-trimester pregnancy loss could have their case histories and notes reviewed to allow certain procedures to be planned, eg cervical cerclage. There is evidence that in properly selected cases, cervical cerclage early in the second trimester reduces the risk of subsequent late miscarriage and early preterm delivery.

For women with a psychiatric history, assessment of their current status may be arranged and reassurance given about the terato-genicity of their drugs. A social network may be set up well in advance, involving the community psychiatric nurse, the GP and social worker, to support the couple during and after pregnancy.

Essay 16

Critically debate the value of prepregnancy clinics.

Essay tips

This question may seem daunting at the outset. It comes in different guises addressing aspects of new, dedicated or managed services in obstetric and gynaecology practice, including: early pregnancy assessment units (EPAU), day assessment units (DAU), antenatal beds and prepregnancy clinics. There are five key areas that merit attention:

1 The patient: her partner and her family – transport, reassurance and counselling
2 The NHS: the money provider, cost implications, money saving, bed/staff savings
3 Hospital doctors: the need to allocate time, consultant input and teaching for juniors
4 The primary care team: midwives, GPs and possible referral and learning opportunity
5 Research, guidelines and audit: these are an absolute must when answering this type of question.

An easy essay plan is shown in the figure:

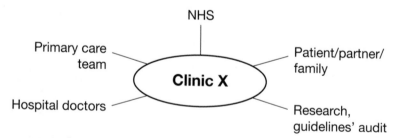

The key words in this question are:

• critically debate
• the value of prepregnancy clinics.

Critically debate

The approach to this type of question and its scope are covered in the introductory section. For example, the NHS has to provide senior staff – including obstetricians, midwives, physicians, geneticists – which costs money. GPs and community midwives should be provided with referral guidelines/protocols so that clinics are run effectively and misuse avoided, eg as a cervical smear clinic. Continuous research and audit are necessary to ensure a high standard.

The value of prepregnancy clinics

If a prepregnancy clinic was cheap and easy to arrange and had a huge benefit for mother and child, we would have these clinics in each and every district and cottage hospital like a gynae or antenatal clinic. But we haven't! There are a number of difficulties, one being the lack of robust evidence to support the benefits of these clinics. There are also funding and staffing problems. Therefore prepregnancy clinics need to be neither praised nor smashed to smithereens. The candidate is required to explore the potential benefits and problems of such clinics.

The essay itself

Prepregnancy clinics aim to reduce maternal and perinatal morbidity and mortality.

Counselling could be offered to patients and their partners, for example for genetic disorders. Adjustments in drug regimens could reduce the risks of fetal malformation, and patients with severe medical disorders could have their condition reviewed with a view to their suitability for pregnancy and timely conception. Women with a complicated obstetric history could be advised to attend a tertiary centre for antenatal care and the previous case notes reviewed and updated. However, awaiting test results, for example for genetic carrier status, may be a psychological burden for couples.

The NHS has to provide senior staff, for example obstetricians, geneticists and counsellors, all of whom have cost implications. Hospital doctors need to be allocated time and be released from other service commitments with potential impact on those services.

Consultant input in the clinic is vital to maintain a strategic direction and high quality care. For junior doctors these clinics could provide a teaching and learning opportunity.

The primary care team (PCT) would have a referral and learning benefit, and therefore could be closely involved into future pregnancy management. This would most probably meet the woman's needs, since it avoids cumbersome travelling and is less time-consuming. However, the PCT needs to be provided with strict referral protocols/guidelines in order to run the clinic effectively and avoid misuse. Continuous research and audit are necessary to ensure a high standard.

Essay 17

A 32-year-old woman attends the antenatal clinic. She is known to be HIV-positive. She is now 14 weeks' pregnant and wishes to discuss the implications of HIV in pregnancy.

How would you counsel her?

Essay tips

The key words in this question are:

- 14 weeks' pregnant
- wishes to discuss
- implications of HIV in pregnancy
- how would you counsel her?

These statements introduce you to the scenario. She is 32 years of age, known to be HIV-positive and attending the antenatal clinic. This background information should be explored further. How advanced is her disease? This can be assessed from laboratory results of her recent viral load and CD4 counts. Is she on any anti-retroviral agents, if so which ones?

14 weeks' pregnant

This gestation is sufficiently early for a safe termination of pregnancy if she requests it. In the past, this was the recommended gestation to commence zidovudine if she wished to proceed with the pregnancy.

Wishes to discuss

The candidate has to work out the most relevant issues that the patient would like to discuss and the likely questions that she would like answered. The counselling should be non-directive. She should be given information on the implications of HIV in pregnancy in a non-judgemental and balanced way. Her concerns might centre on the following questions:

- Will my baby be normal?
- Will my baby have AIDS?
- Is there anything I can do?
- Will the disease break out in pregnancy?
- etc, etc.

Implications of HIV in pregnancy

This is the main part of your essay. Since knowledge in this area is continually advancing and changing, a good candidate should be familiar with the current guidelines and publications on HIV in pregnancy. The implications may be divided into those for the mother and those for the fetus/neonate.

Maternal	Fetal/Neonatal
Markers of disease progression not adversely affected by pregnancy	The rate of vertical transmission is approximately 15% without intervention (25% in Africa)
Lower transmission rate with: • high levels of anti-HIV • antibodies • low viral load • avoidance of breast-feeding • delivery by Caesarean section • antiretroviral agents	No more adverse fetal effects than in an HIV negative pregnancy No practical methods of prenatal diagnosis to predict which infants are affected
Higher transmission rate with: • P24 antigenaemia • CD4 count $<$ 200/mm • prematurity $<$ 34 weeks' gestation • high viral load Invasive prenatal diagnosis should be avoided	Most neonatal infections occur during delivery Early diagnosis of HIV infection in the neonate may also be difficult because of persisting maternal antibodies for up to 18 months. This is now less of a problem with the application of DNA amplification techniques

How would you counsel her?

Mentioning allocation of time and senior staff to the patient and her partner might carry a mark. You would ensure the counselling took place in a private area, with no outside interruptions. Sometimes, but not always, the RCOG awards marks for a well-planned and rounded essay. Nevertheless, the overall balance of an essay that includes all aspects of clinical care is much better, and the examiner might be willing to award you an extra mark elsewhere!

The essay itself

A senior member of staff should counsel this woman in an atmosphere of privacy, with time allocated for it. Preferably, her partner should be present during the discussion and a sympathetic approach adopted.

Information to impart during counselling

Markers of disease progression in the mother are not adversely affected by pregnancy, but despite this she may opt for termination of the pregnancy because of concerns for the unborn child and her own perceived reduced life expectancy.

Although the transmission rate to the fetus is about 15%, this can be lowered to about 1–2% with a package of interventions including antenatal antiretroviral medication, elective Caesarean section, bottle-feeding rather than breast-feeding and neonatal antiretroviral agents. Higher transmission rates are found in patients with high viral loads, P24 antigenaemia, low CD4 counts < 200/ml and in premature deliveries < 34 weeks. If the woman is already on the triple regimen of 'highly active antiretroviral therapy' (HAART) her viral load may be undetectable and, at least theoretically, there is a negligible risk of vertical transmission to the fetus. There is some suggestion that an elective Caesarean section may not offer additional benefit for the fetus. On the other hand, there is scanty data on viral shedding into genital-tract secretions of women with an undetectable viral load in their serum. Vaginal delivery in this situation is best agreed on an individual patient basis.

Methods of invasive prenatal diagnosis should be avoided, and detailed ultrasound based screening used. With respect to the fetus, there are no more adverse effects than in HIV-negative pregnancies. However, there are no practical methods of prenatal diagnosis to predict which infants are/will be infected. Most neonatal infections occur during the perinatal period, which is the justification for the Caesarean section. The difficulty associated with early neonatal HIV diagnosis is now being overcome by the introduction of DNA-amplification testing such as PCR (polymerase chain reaction) rather than reliance on antibody assays. Maternal antibodies may persist for up to 18 months and IgM antibodies are unhelpful in fetal diagnosis. Joint obstetric care with HIV physicians should be arranged and booking under a consultant organised.

At present, azidothymidine (AZT; zidovudine) is the only antiretroviral agent licensed for use during pregnancy in the UK. It has a relatively long track record of use in the perinatal period and carries a small risk of neonatal mitochondrial dysfunction. There are no long-term safety data on infants and children exposed to other antiretroviral agents.

Essay 18

A 26-year-old primigravida is admitted at 27 weeks' gestation, semi-conscious and with a history of convulsions.

Outline the possible causes and principles of management.

Essay tips
The key words in this question are:

- 26-year-old primigravida
- admitted
- semi-conscious
- 27 weeks' gestation
- outline
- possible causes
- principles of management.

26-year-old primigravida
She is of average age, but more importantly she is primigravid. In this scenario, consideration must be given to the possibility of an eclamptic fit, but by no means is this the entire story.

Admitted
She is in the hospital (not in the community, for example). Therefore advice and input from other colleagues and specialists is available. This implies that a multidisciplinary team approach can be adopted and arrangements made for intensive or high-dependency care.

Semi-conscious
'Semi-conscious' suggests she might be able to provide some basic history/information. Other relevant history may be extracted from her clinical records, the community midwife/GP or any referring person as well as her family or partner.

27 weeks' gestation
The fetus is very premature at this gestation. Delivery in the interest of the mother is a crucial decision, but, first, the correct diagnosis has to be established. At 27 weeks' gestation, senior

paediatric input and steroid administration should be considered while maternal resuscitation and stabilisation are ongoing. When this is achieved and delivery is judged to be necessary, arrangements can be initiated for transfer to a larger unit, either *in utero* if the mother is stable and it is appropriate, or *ex utero*.

Outline

'Outline' means stating the main facts or points required without elaborating, explaining or justifying them.

Possible causes

The possible causes might be related or unrelated to pregnancy.

- Pregnancy-related include:
    - eclampsia
    - gestational epilepsy.

- Unrelated to pregnancy are:
    - cerebral vein thrombosis (CVT)
    - cerebral infarction
    - thrombotic thrombocytopenic purpura (TTP)
    - drug and alcohol withdrawal
    - metabolic causes
        - hypoglycaemia
        - hypocalcaemia
        - hyponatraemia
    - epilepsy, and
    - pseudoepilepsy.

Note that nobody has said this woman has eclampsia. She is semi-conscious after a convulsion. That is all we know! It is up to the candidate to suggest the possible reasons why this may have happened.

Principles of management

The College is quite fond of this phrase. This is a management question, and therefore requires comments on the history and examination of this patient, investigations, treatment and follow-up.

When dealing with obstetric emergencies the principles of management are, relatively speaking, almost constant, namely:

- resuscitation
- communication
- monitoring
- investigating, and
- treating synchronously.

An opening sentence incorporating this list gives the immediate impression that the candidate is a safe doctor with a sound knowledge base and is likely to have dealt with situations like this before.

- **Resuscitation**: position the patient; clear the airway and provide an oxygen supply; insert two intravenous access lines and start a drip, etc. Also organise an ITU/HDU bed.

- **Communication**: extract a history from her notes; ask the patient, partner, or whoever has accompanied her to hospital for any information; and also involve the midwife, senior obstetrician, anaesthetist, physician, porter, haematologist, etc.

- **Monitoring**: for vital signs (BP, pulse, RR), ECG, blood results, urinary output and constituents, CVP as necessary.

- **Investigations**: request a FBC (including platelet count and a blood film for a differential count) and clotting screen, U&E, liver function tests, uric acid, blood glucose, urinalysis, drug levels, calcium, sodium as well as CT/MRI scans, EEG and, lastly, fetal heart investigations.

- **Treatment**: this will depend on the underlying cause.

The essay itself

As in any obstetric emergency, the cause(s) may be related or unrelated to pregnancy. While eclampsia and gestational epilepsy are unique to pregnancy, convulsions can also be caused by cerebral vein thrombosis (CVT), cerebral infarction, thrombotic thrombocytopenic purpura (TTP), drug and alcohol withdrawal, metabolic disorders, eg hypoglycaemia, hypocalcaemia and hyponatraemia. Convulsions can also be due to epilepsy or pseudoepilepsy occurring during pregnancy.

The principles of management include resuscitation undertaken simultaneously, communication, monitoring, investigation and treatment of the patient.

Immediate management

Resuscitation of this semi-conscious patient begins with the appropriate positioning, clearance of the airway as needed, and provision of an oxygen supply. Two large cannulas should be sited to secure venous access for fluid replacement and medications.

A multidisciplinary team approach involving senior obstetricians, anaesthetists, physicians, paediatricians, porters and haematologists should be assembled and a bed in the high-dependency unit organised.

History

Communication is vital. A history from the patient herself, her notes, the referring healthcare worker, her partner, family or friend should be extracted. Important questions are whether this is the first episode, presence of any prodromal symptoms, headache, restlessness, visual disturbance, and also a history of drug or alcohol abuse, diabetes, hypoadrenalism, hypopituitarism, liver failure, epilepsy or hypoparathyroidism.

Examination

A full, general and neurological examination should be performed, including a check for papillary oedema, neck stiffness and reflexes/clonus.

Vital signs should be monitored frequently, eg every 15–30 minutes initially, including blood pressure and pulse rate. Frequently monitor her ECG, blood results, urinary output, central venous pressure and blood glucose levels.

Investigations

These will include a full blood count (including a platelet count and blood film for a differential count) and clotting screen, U&E, liver function tests, uric acid, blood glucose, calcium, sodium, drug levels as indicated, and urinalysis. A CT/MRI scan and EEG may be indicated and the fetal heart rate should also be monitored.

Treatment

Treatment will depend on the underlying cause, but the priority is to stabilise the patient. Magnesium sulphate and antihypertensives are given in cases of eclampsia. Steroids should be given, and the infant delivered regardless of its prematurity. Transport arrangements to a tertiary referral centre may be necessary. Treatment of CVT is with anticonvulsants, as for epilepsy, but the use of heparin is debatable. TTP can be treated with fresh-frozen plasma, and plasmapheresis and corticosteroids may be of benefit. Platelet replacement should be avoided in patients with TTP. Drug and alcohol abuse is best treated in close liaison with the psychiatrist. In a diabetic patient, use of a sliding scale will help in the correction of blood sugar levels. Hypoglycaemia may be corrected with glucagon in an emergency. Other metabolic deficiencies can be corrected by delivery of the appropriate treatment through an infusion pump under close supervision and with the involvement of specialist physicians.

Follow-up

Follow-up arrangements are essential after resolution of the acute phase.

Essay 19

A 45-year-old grand-multiparous woman presents at 7 weeks' gestation in the antenatal booking clinic.

Formulate a management plan specific to her pregnancy.

Essay tips

The key words in this question are:

- 45-year-old – pregnant
- grand-multiparous
- 7 weeks' gestation
- antenatal booking clinic
- formulate a management plan
- specific.

45-year-old – pregnant

Consider the influence of maternal age on this pregnancy and the effect of pregnancy on a woman of this age. What features would be more or less common compared to those in a 25-year-old pregnant woman? See the essay plan on the next page.

There is an increased risk of pregnancy complications, including miscarriage and multiple pregnancy during the first trimester. An early ultrasound scan is therefore indicated. Fibroids and ovarian cysts may be incidental findings, the former being more common in this age group. Because a woman of this age has a 1:50 risk of having a fetus with chromosomal abnormality such as a Down syndrome, she may opt to have a nuchal translucency test, a triple test or a direct, invasive, prenatal diagnostic test. Explore the mother's past obstetric history and review her notes. Hypertensive disorders are more common and so is gestational diabetes. Arrangements for regular blood pressure checks and a glucose tolerance test (GTT) need to be mapped out. Underlying medical disorders may already antedate this pregnancy, for example essential hypertension or diabetes mellitus. Existing drug regimens may need to be changed to ones that are suitable for use in pregnancy. Close liaison with the physicians and booking under consultant care is certainly justified in a woman of this age.

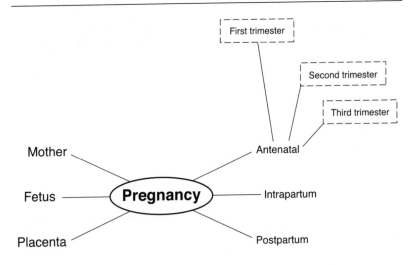

Candidates who run out of time may consider a brief summary using bullet points:

- First trimester:
  - increased risk of miscarriage, ectopic/molar/multiple pregnancy
  - screening for Down syndrome using nuchal translucency
  - ? early CVS.

- Second trimester:
  - screening for Down syndrome (triple test, CVS, amniocentesis)
  - fetal abnormality scan
  - start growth scan, cave IUGR
  - increased risk of antepartum haemorrhage
  - correct anaemia in pregnancy.

- Third trimester:
  - fetal surveillance (USS, BPP, Doppler)
  - a plan for an earlier delivery may become necessary, for example induction of labour preterm, if the tests detect abnormalities.

- Intrapartum:
  - ensure iv access, request a full blood count and 'Group and save' for the increased risk of operative delivery and possible anaemia and postpartum haemorrhage. Grand multiparity on its own is not associated with PPH.

- partogram – the pelvic soft tissues may be more rigid due to the mother's age, and dystocia may occur even after previous normal deliveries.

- Postpartum:
  - thromboprophylaxis
  - contraception.

- Maternal:
  - increased risk of medical disorders, eg essential hypertension
  - increased incidence of coexistent gynaecological problems interfering with the pregnancy – such as fibroids
  - increased incidence of pregnancy-induced hypertension and gestational diabetes, regular BP, urine checks and a GTT advised
  - increased risk of thromboembolism therefore provide prophylaxis.

- Fetal:
  - increased risk of chromosomal abnormalities, dizygotic twins and IUGR.

- Placental:
  - increased risk of placenta praevia.

Grand-multiparous

She has delivered at least four children and she may be anaemic especially if the deliveries were at short intervals. Multiparity combined with advanced maternal age puts this patient at an increased risk of placenta praevia. Further associated problems include malpresentation and an unstable lie towards term, which may lead to the need for hospitalisation and disruption of her domestic arrangement. The third stage of labour should be managed actively because of the increased risk of postpartum haemorrhage. However, an ergometrine and oxytocin preparation (Syntometrine) should be used with caution if she has coexistent hypertensive disease. This woman is also at an increased risk of atypical blood antibodies and due attention should be paid to this if blood products are required.

7 weeks' gestation

The College wants a full overview of the entire pregnancy, which is why this early gestational age is chosen. Do not assume a viable, single intrauterine pregnancy. This has not been stated. You will lose valuable marks if you make such an assumption.

Antenatal booking clinic

Booking investigations, including scans, have to be mentioned, but do not list all the tests, for example: syphilis, rubella, etc. 'Routine booking investigations' is the phrase to use, then 'Special attention should be paid to...' once you talk about, let's say, an ultrasound scan or haemoglobin level.

Formulate a management plan

A management plan is slightly different to management alone. The information needs to be placed in specific sections, as the figure of the essay plan suggests. The plan should be communicated to the woman in a non-directive manner, with sufficient flexibility to accommodate her wishes and choice. History, examination and investigations leading to proper treatment are still required in the answer, albeit not in a rigidly structured way.

Specific

Specific' means 'specific'! No waffle! The candidate should restrict him/herself to the essentials: age-related pregnancy problems and grand-multiparity.

The essay itself

Advanced maternal age and grand-multiparity combine to make this a high-risk pregnancy. Therefore consultant-led care is more appropriate, with multidisciplinary input as required.

First trimester

Miscarriage, ectopic/molar/multiple pregnancies and uterine fibroids are not uncommon during the first trimester.

Routine booking investigations should be performed, with particular attention paid to her haemoglobin level as there is a likelihood of anaemia. Atypical antibodies are more common, and a careful past medical, drug and obstetric history should be obtained since underlying medical disorders are more likely in this age group. A booking scan by an experienced sonographer should be considered and pregnancy dates confirmed and documented.

As the risk of Down's syndrome is 1:50, a screening test (in the form of nuchal translucency measurement) may be offered after careful counselling. She may opt for invasive prenatal diagnosis to establish the fetal karyotype and therefore appropriate referrals should be made.

Second trimester

Iron supplementation should be given if appropriate, and folic acid may be continued throughout the pregnancy.

Antepartum haemorrhage and placenta praevia are common in women of this age. Since hypertensive disorders and gestational diabetes are also more common in older pregnant women, regular blood pressure and urine checks and a glucose tolerance test should be considered, especially if there is a glycosuria or large for gestational age fetus.

A fetal anomaly scan should be offered at 20–22 weeks' gestation. The fetus is at a higher risk of intrauterine growth restriction and close surveillance is required, including an ultrasound scan for fetal growth, a biophysical profile, Doppler and CTG assessments for indicators of fetal compromise.

Third trimester and intrapartum

An abnormal placental location/praevia should be excluded during the third trimester, especially if there is malposition or vaginal bleeding. There is a higher risk of a malpresentation and unstable lie of the fetus necessitating admission towards term, which may be socially disruptive to the family. Therefore a good supporting social network needs to be in place. Consider involving social services.

Spontaneous vaginal delivery should be anticipated, but a caesarean delivery should be planned if there are other obstetric indications. Thromboprophylaxis is indicated whether delivery is by Caesarean section or not. There is no specific increase in the risk of postpartum haemorrhage (PPH) but an iv line, full blood count and 'Group and save' may be required because of the higher risk of operative delivery.

A partogram should be followed and abnormal patterns of labour recognised and treated early. If required, the use of oxytocin should be sanctioned by a senior obstetrician, applied sparingly and with great caution because of the increased risk of uterine rupture. The third stage of labour should be managed actively to reduce the risk of PPH, but an ergot based preparation (eg Syntometrine) would be contraindicated in the presence of hypertensive disorders. Such women should be treated with five units of Syntometrine.

Postpartum

A detailed discussion of contraception is needed during the post-partum period and, if necessary, continued social support organised for the mother and her family.

Essay 20

A multiparous woman despite having good uterine contractions remains in the second stage of labour for two hours. At pelvic examination the fetal head is found to be in the occipitotransverse position.

Justify your decision on the mode of delivery.

Essay tips
The key words in this question are

- multiparous
- good uterine contractions
- 2 hours in the second stage
- pelvic examination
- occipitotransverse position
- justify your decision
- mode of delivery.

Multiparous
As this woman has a past obstetric history, details of her previous delivery/deliveries, especially if delivery was by Caesarean section, should be sought. What stage of labour (if unplanned) did this occur, was the onset of labour spontaneous or induced, was regional analgesia used and what were the sizes of the babies. These considerations are important when it comes to justifying your actions.

Good uterine contractions
Note that she is multiparous. The use of oxytocin in this situation carries a risk of uterine rupture. Although approximately 8% of multiparous women will have dysfunctional uterine action, especially if there is a long gap after their last delivery, the contractions in this case are described as 'good'. Further stimulation is unlikely to be of benefit. In general, if oxytocin is considered in such a case, it must be approved by a senior obstetrician, who should exclude mechanical obstruction and ensure that oxytocin is used sparingly and monitored very closely.

Two hours in the second stage

Two hours in the second stage of labour is excessively long for a parous woman unless she has epidural analgesia. There is no advantage in leaving her any longer. Prompt assessment and a clear management plan are needed. The partogram, CTG and state of the amniotic fluid should be reviewed. The abdomen should be examined to assess the stage of descent/engagement of the head.

Pelvic examination

A thorough clinical assessment should be undertaken of the adequacy of the bony pelvis and the soft tissues relative to the size of the baby. The station of the vertex in relation to the ischial spines should be determined. The presence and severity of caput and moulding should be documented, as well as the degree of deflection of the fetal head and asynclitism.

Occipitotransverse position (OT)

In cases of malposition of the fetal head, you need a senior obstetrician and appropriate analgesia for the woman. You should also consider undertaking the delivery in theatre.

Justify your decision

Why would you make what decision? The candidate should describe different scenarios after introducing the examiner to his/her considerations as highlighted above.

Examples

- If this woman had had a previous Caesarean section and more than one-fifth of the baby's head was palpable per abdomen in addition to significant caput and moulding, a Caesarean section would be the safer option for mother and child.

- If she has a capacious pelvis and an average-sized fetus, manual rotation may be attempted and delivery completed with a vacuum cup; alternatively she could have a low-cavity forceps delivery.

- In low transverse arrest, a posterior vacuum cup may be applied. This has the ability to achieve autorotation with traction. An alternative approach is the application of Kielland's rotational forceps if the operator has the expertise and is sufficiently experienced.

Mode of delivery

The woman/partner should be involved in the decision-making process with regard to the mode of delivery. A spontaneous vaginal delivery is unlikely to be successful in this scenario, and there are inherent risks in persisting with this option. That leaves you with two options: instrumental vaginal delivery and emergency Caesarean section. This question is not about whether vacuum is better than forceps, the spectrum is much broader. An emergency Caesarean section at full cervical dilatation is technically difficult, so a senior obstetrician is needed.

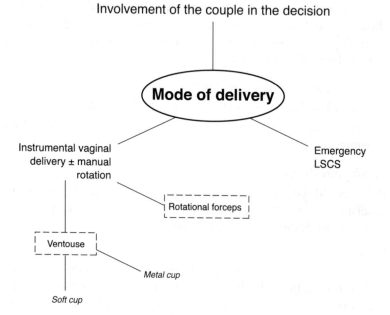

The essay itself

Management of a delay in the second stage of labour in a parous woman should be handled or directly supervised by a senior obstetrician to ensure a satisfactory outcome.

The woman's past obstetric history should be obtained and further information gleaned from the clinical notes, especially relating to the modes of deliveries, sizes of the babies and their gestations at delivery.

An abdominal examination should be undertaken, to determine the degree of the fetal head engagement and to give a rough estimate of fetal size and state of the bladder. Prior to pelvic examination, a vulval oedema might be noted and the colour of liquor appraised. At pelvic examination, the capacity of the pelvis, the station of the fetal head, presence and severity of caput and moulding are all assessed. Some deflexion of the head might be present.

Fetal wellbeing should be established by continuous CTG monitoring and the partogram reviewed.

Expectant management is unlikely to lead to a normal vaginal delivery, and poses several potential hazards for the mother, including uterine rupture, fistula formation, long-term pelvic dysfunction, postpartum haemorrhage and fetal distress. Oxytocin in the presence of good uterine activity in a parous labour is inappropriate, and increases the risk of uterine rupture with the further potential for fetomaternal morbidity and mortality.

The options lie between an instrumental vaginal delivery and an emergency Caesarean section. Patient consent, transfer to theatre and appropriate analgesia given by a senior anaesthetist are all essential. In either case, the mother and her partner should be involved in the decision.

Rotation of the head and vaginal delivery may be attempted in a non-distressed fetus with the vertex at or below the ischial spines, and without significant caput and/or moulding. Manual rotation and the application of a silastic vacuum cup is a reasonable course of action in a parous woman with a capacious pelvis and an average-sized fetus, and is associated with fewer fetal scalp injuries. A low cavity forceps delivery is an alternative. A posterior metal vacuum cup may also be applied and autorotation achieved during traction. However, metal cups are associated with more scalp injuries. The Kielland's forceps in experienced hands may be used to rotate and complete delivery of the infant. There is, however, a higher risk of maternal genital tract trauma and postpartum haemorrhage. It should be borne in mind that any rotation manoeuvre carries a risk of cord prolapse.

An emergency Caesarean section should be undertaken if there are signs of obstruction to progress during the second stage of labour. For instance, where more than one-fifth of the fetal head is palpable per abdomen and/or the vertex is above the level of the ischial spines; and where there is significant caput, moulding and deflexion of the fetal head, with or without fetal distress. This is the preferred and safer option for mother and child, and also applies if she has had a previous Caesarean section. However, an emergency Caesarean section under these circumstances is hazardous, with the attendant risks of: injury to the bladder; postpartum haemorrhage due to the extension of the uterotomy angles intraoperatively; infection and thromboembolism postoperatively. A senior obstetrician should be involved and antibiotic/thromboprophylaxis implemented.

Essay 21

Compare and contrast the different drugs available for thromboprophylaxis in pregnancy.

Essay tips
The key words in this question are:

- compare and contrast
- different drugs
- available
- prophylaxis
- thromboprophylaxis in pregnancy.

Compare and contrast
This question requires you to present the similarities and differences of various classes of drugs available for thromboprophylaxis in pregnancy. For example, summarise the characteristics of those administered orally versus those given parenterally, those that cross the placenta and the ones that do not. This is the comparing part. In contrasting them, the differences are presented, for example, aspirin and warfarin can both be conveniently administered orally, but significant teratogenicity is only known for warfarin.

Different drugs
Drugs available for thromboprophylaxis during pregnancy include aspirin, warfarin and heparin, both unfractionated (sometimes called 'standard') and low molecular weight formulations. You may wish to mention the outdated dextran, only to condemn it again. Occasionally, the College awards an extra mark for such excursions into obstetric history!

Of interest in this question are issues like:

- routes of administration
- maternal side-effects
- teratogenicity/fetal side-effects
- the need to monitor clotting parameters
- reversibility.

There should be no reference to anti-TED (thromboembolic disease) stockings. Only drugs have been asked for!

Available

Remember that your local protocol and hospital formulary may not contain all the drugs available for this indication. Therefore you need to think widely and laterally for the information you require to answer the question satisfactorily.

Prophylaxis

This question is about prevention of thromboembolism not the treatment of it.

Thromboprophylaxis in pregnancy

Pregnant women should be classified into the following thromboembolic risk groups:

- low
- medium
- high risk.

A clear knowledge of who should be included in which group will be useful in answering this question. For the second triennium running, thromboembolism is the leading cause of direct maternal mortality in the UK and is a 'hot' membership essay question.

Pregnancy

Remember antenatal, intrapartum and postpartum.

The essay itself

Thromboembolism is the leading cause of maternal mortality in the UK and its prevention is a key objective in perinatal care. Since any drug treatment has the potential of producing unwanted side-effects, a risk assessment of the pregnant woman should first be undertaken.

Aspirin can be administered orally in a once-daily dose of 75 mg. The results of randomised trials have shown it to be effective in reducing the risk of thrombosis in medical and surgical patients, but the evidence for its efficacy in pregnancy is less robust. However, it has been shown to be safe in observational studies. There is no risk of teratogenicity nor is there any need to monitor blood levels; and the risk of maternal gastrointestinal bleeding is very small. Its place is in the prevention of antenatal thromboembolism in women at low risk, such as those with a single previous thromboembolic event and without other risk factors.

Heparin has to be administered via subcutaneous injection and compliance may be a problem. It has the advantage of not crossing the placenta and therefore has no adverse effects on the fetus. However, thrombocytopenia – especially the idiosyncratic immune-mediated variety occurring 6–10 days after the commencement of prophylaxis – is rare but potentially life-threatening. Although the early form of thrombocytopenia is relatively harmless, initial weekly platelet counts are recommended. Osteoporosis is another side-effect, especially with long-term heparin use, but fortunately it is reversible.

Low molecular weight heparin (LMWH) has a higher bioavailability and potentially better side-effect profile than unfractionated heparin, and can therefore be given once daily. It is given to low-risk women intrapartum and postpartum as an alternative to warfarin. High-risk women – for example, those with thrombophilia, a family history of thromboembolism, recurrent thromboembolism in the current pregnancy – also receive heparin antenatally. Its drug effect can be speedily reversed if needed by protamine sulphate.

Warfarin can be given orally but it crosses the placenta and has a well-documented teratogenic effect, the risk of which is approximately 5%. It should be avoided in the first trimester altogether, and its tendency to cause microcephaly and neurological abnormalities in fetuses exposed during the second trimester is well described. Beyond 36 weeks' gestation, retroplacental and intracerebral bleeding are reported. Close monitoring of the INR is necessary so the dose of warfarin can be adjusted. The effects can be reversed by the administration of fresh-frozen plasma and a host of newer but expensive agents. In the light of this its use during the antenatal period is restricted to women with metal heart valves whose thromboembolic risk is high. However, warfarin can be used for postnatal prophylaxis for women in all risk categories for 6 weeks.

Dextran has been used in the past, but it interferes with maternal blood grouping and has therefore been abandoned.

Essay 22

Describe the complications of Caesarean section and discuss the possible methods of prevention.

Essay tips

The key words in this question are:

- describe
- complications
- Caesarean section
- discuss
- methods of prevention.

Describe

A description is something you provide for someone else's understanding. The task is to make the examiner understand exactly what you are describing. Therefore avoid long, convoluted and waffling statements.

Complications

Structure these into short-term and long-term complications. Complications may be due to the actions of a surgeon or the characteristics of the patient. (Of course, at the end of the day it is always the surgeon!) Furthermore, consider the intra- and postoperative complications, as well as policy actions that will reduce the risk of complications occurring such as application/adherence to protocols/guidelines and audit activities.

Caesarean section

Although all surgical procedures carry a risk of haemorrhage, infection and thromboembolism, these risks are higher with Caesarean section. This is because the procedure involves a very vascular uterus at term and its placental bed. The operating field is in direct communication with the vagina. Furthermore pregnancy is a thrombogenic state. From the surgeon's standpoint, a detailed knowledge of the fetomaternal history, examination findings and investigation results are essential. Training, appropriate experience and senior input at the right time saves lives and prevents litigations.

135

Discuss

What can be done and how can these be done to prevent the complications of Caesarean section. In a discussion essay, consideration should be given to all the controversies, cost implications, potential harm/benefits and effectiveness of the interventions as well as the steps proposed, including the evidence (or lack of it) to back them up.

Methods of prevention

There are two possible approaches to this essay: the candidate may write down the complications in the first part and match them with the preventive measures in the second part, or combine these two parts and discuss them in pairs in prose style. The author's suggestion is that the latter option saves time, provided you have a good essay plan (opposite).

Complications	Protocols, audit, re-audit	Prevention
Lack of experience; excessive speed	**Surgeons**	Training; senior input
Special circumstances, eg previous PPH, obesity, placenta praevia and previous Caesarean section	**Patients**	Knowledge of history, examination and investigation results of both mother and fetus
Ruptured membranes; < 32/40 weeks' gestation; low vertex; haemorrhage; extension into broad ligament	**Intraoperative**	Senior input Deliver head OA Crossmatch; anticipate need for hysterectomy
Thromboembolism Infection UTI Wound Wound dehiscence	**Postoperative: short term**	Risk assessment for all patients Antibiotics for all patients In-and-out catheter only Good surgical technique Mass closure for patients at risk Wound drains
Reduced chance of vaginal delivery	**Postoperative: long term**	Consider appropriateness of Caesarean section in the first instance

The essay itself

The complications of Caesarean sections may be avoided by the early recognition of risk factors, for example: delivery before 32 weeks' gestation; ruptured membranes; and deeply engaged vertex. Lack of experience and expertise on the part of the surgeon are additional factors. Therefore, from the surgeons' perspective, good training, knowledge of the history, examination and investigation results of both mother and child are paramount, as well as well-timed senior input.

Haemorrhage might occur intra- and postoperatively. In women who have had a previous Caesarean section, a preoperative scan may detect placenta praevia. Therefore precautions can be taken to prevent the massive haemorrhage and its complications, including, crossmatching blood and ensuring the presence of a senior obstetrician and anaesthetist. This also applies to patients with a previous postpartum haemorrhage, obesity, prolonged second stage labour, pre-eclampsia, amnionitis and when a classical Caesarean section is anticipated. In some circumstances, hysterectomy may be anticipated and the surgeon should be familiar with the variety of techniques to avoid this, for example a B-Lynch brace suture. Wide lateral dissection of the bladder should be avoided to prevent tears in the broad ligament and, for the same reason, the fetal head should be delivered in the occipitoanterior (OA) position. The skin incision should be no less than 15 cm. Traditionally a continuous, locking, double-layer suture with Vicryl is used for uterine closure. Trials are in progress comparing this to single-layer closure. Non-closure of the peritoneum helps a quicker return of bowel sounds and is associated with less infectious morbidity.

Routine prophylactic, broad-spectrum antibiotics reduces the risk of postoperative infection. Once-only catheterisation immediately preoperatively helps to avoid urinary tract infection, although urinary retention due to regional block and postoperative pain nullifies this advantage. Good surgical technique, secure haemostasis and wound drainage all help to reduce the risk of wound infection and wound breakdown. The rectus sheath should be closed with large bites using robust suture materials. For patients at high risk of postoperative dehiscence, mass closure using the Smeade–Jones technique and polydioxanone suture (PDS) material should be considered.

Thromboembolism is closely related to Caesarean sections and a risk assessment for all women followed by appropriate prophylaxis, including the use of TED stockings and heparin, is mandatory. The early mobilisation and discharge of women with straightforward operations may help to avoid nosocomial infections. In the long term the woman's chance of vaginal delivery is reduced. Therefore the appropriateness of Caesarean delivery needs to be assured in the first instance, and a trial of labour offered whenever possible and agreeable with the woman. Protocols and guidelines should be available to prevent complications at Caesarean sections, and regular audit and re-audit performed to ensure that high standards are continuously maintained.

Essay 23

A 29-year-old primigravid woman presents at 28 weeks' gestation with a marked oligohydramnios.

Justify your investigations.

Essay tips

The key words in this question are:

- 29-year-old
- primigravid
- marked oligohydramnios
- justify
- investigations.

29-year-old

She may have an antecedent medical history, which could relate to the oligohydramnios. The history might include a chronic illness, drugs like indometacin and heavy cigarette smoking.

Primigravid

Pre-eclampsia is more common in this group and should form part of your investigations.

Marked oligohydramnios

The causes of perinatal problems could be:

- maternal
- fetal
- placental.

Intrauterine growth retardation (IUGR) may be the commonest cause, but certainly not the only one. The candidate should consider the differential diagnosis of oligohydramnios and not suggest a Doppler ultrasound scan examination as the only relevant investigation. Preterm, prelabour rupture of membranes (PPROM) should also be considered.

	Maternal	Fetal	Placental
Possible causes	Smoking Drugs, eg indomethacin PET PPROM	Malformation, esp. renal tract or others, eg hypoplastic lungs IUD, IUGR	Insufficiency
Investigations	Review MSAFP 24-h urine collection for protein PET bloods Speculum exam, nitrazine and ferning tests, scan	Scan for viability and fetal abnormalities Doppler of mid-cerebral artery Growth scan ?Invasive prenatal diagnostic test(s)	Doppler scan of umbilical artery

Abbreviations: PET, pre-eclamptic toxaemia; PPROM, preterm, prelabour rupture of membranes; IUD, intrauterine death; IUGR, intrauterine growth retardation; MSAFP, maternal serum α-fetoprotein.

Justify

Why would you do what investigation? Which tests are appropriate in evaluating severe oligohydramnios? Remember that these tests should be directed at the mother, the fetus and the placenta.

Investigations

Appropriate investigations are usually based on the history and examination findings. The difference here is that this patient has presented with the result of investigation. Consider you are the specialist registrar in the antenatal clinic and have been asked to see this woman who has just returned from the ultrasound scan department with this report. What other tests might you request, and why, to help you characterise the cause of the oligohydramnios?

The essay itself

'Marked oligohydramnios' describes the situation whereby the largest vertical pocket of amniotic fluid is considerably less than 2 cm. It is associated with a 40-fold increase in the perinatal mortality rate. The causes may be maternal, fetal or placental.

A maternal history of heavy smoking and/or therapy with drugs that may reduce the amniotic fluid volume (eg indometacin) should be explored. Any history of a sudden loss/gush of fluid or a persistent and uncontrollable loss from the vagina should be noted. Her early pregnancy biochemical markers such as serum α-fetoprotein (if taken) should be reviewed. Her blood pressure should be checked and a midstream urine sample obtained to check for the presence of protein. If positive, a 24-h urine collection for total protein excretion should be commenced, and blood taken for a full blood count (including a blood film for a differential count), clotting screen, U&E, urate, liver function tests and 'Group and save', since severe pre-eclamptic toxaemia (PET) might be a cause of the oligohydramnios.

A speculum vaginal examination should be performed for the presence of amniotic fluid. The use of the nitrazine pH-based test for amniotic fluid may be used, although false-positive results are common in the presence of vaginitis, blood and semen, and contact with cervical secretions. The fern test may give a false-negative at this stage of gestation.

Placental causes of oligohydramnios include placental insufficiency, and a Doppler waveform analysis of the umbilical artery may show increased resistance to blood flow to the placental bed. In cases of absent or reversed flow, delivery may be indicated despite the early gestational age. However, a delay for 24–48 h should be considered to allow for corticosteroid administration and transfer to a tertiary centre if necessary.

For the diagnosis of IUGR, measurements of the head circumference biparietal diameter, abdominal circumference and femur length should be obtained, and the head-sparing effect would support the diagnosis. Doppler waveform analysis of the middle cerebral artery and ductus venosus would give some additional information on the physiological adaptations and state of compensation. A biophysical profile (BPP), though time-consuming, has its place in the management of high-risk pregnancies and assesses fetal breathing movements, gross body movements, fetal tone and reactivity of the fetal heart rate in addition to CTG and amniotic fluid volumes. A score of four or less would support a decision for preterm delivery. A fetal blood sample may be obtained for karyotyping and analysis of fetal acid–base status, although there is a finite risk of fetal loss that is probably as high as 5–10%. Nevertheless, the information can be utilised to decide when and how to deliver this woman.

Some 70% of cases of marked oligohydramnios may be due to IUGR. Intrauterine death and fetal malformation should also be considered. Therefore, an expert should perform an ultrasound scan to check for fetal viability and to exclude an underlying fetal abnormality. Emphasis should be placed on renal tract agenesis, of which Potter's syndrome is the commonest. Lower urinary tract obstructions/abnormalities and hypoplasia of fetal lungs are other differentials. If there are features suggestive of clinical syndromes, this should be discussed and invasive prenatal diagnosis in the form of amniocentesis or chorionic villus biopsy offered to establish the fetal karyotype. This may help to determine the management of the rest of the pregnancy.

Essay 24

A woman has had a failed trial of rotational forceps delivery and is now prepared to be delivered by emergency Caesarean section.

Give a detailed account of the surgical measures you would implement to ensure a safe delivery.

Essay tips

The key words in this question are:

- the scenario as written in the first sentence
- give a detailed account
- surgical measures
- you

The scenario as written

Failed trial of rotational forceps delivery – emergency Caesarean section in the second stage. A second-stage Caesarean section is a challenging procedure. The mother faces the risks of bladder injury and haemorrhage as well as infection and thromboembolism. The baby's head is probably deeply impacted and in malposition therefore difficult to deliver (otherwise there was no indication for rotational forceps in the first place).

Give a detailed account

This implies that you describe what you do. Instead of writing: 'One green Armitage has to be placed on either angle of the uterotomy, and at least one on the lower segment and bleeding points as they occur…', you could write: 'The uterine angles should be swiftly localised, secured and suture of the uterotomy started to achieve prompt haemostasis.'

Surgical measures

The difficulties mainly arise from a high bladder, a stretched lower segment and vagina, and a deeply impacted fetal head. The question says 'surgical', which restricts your mind pretty much to knife, scissors and toothed forceps, not to what the anaesthetist or the paediatrician has to do. After you have managed this heroic Caesarean section don't forget to check the cervix and vagina from down below! Remember she had a failed rotational forceps delivery, so injuries might have occurred necessitating sutures.

You…

Yes, you!!! This time it is unlikely you would get a mark for calling your consultant.

The figure below may help you to remember the big points of concern and the way out of the crisis.

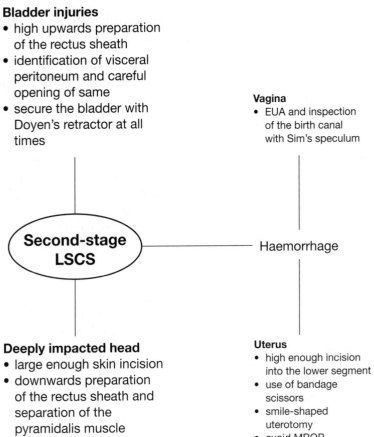

Bladder injuries
- high upwards preparation of the rectus sheath
- identification of visceral peritoneum and careful opening of same
- secure the bladder with Doyen's retractor at all times

Vagina
- EUA and inspection of the birth canal with Sim's speculum

Second-stage LSCS ———————— Haemorrhage

Deeply impacted head
- large enough skin incision
- downwards preparation of the rectus sheath and separation of the pyramidalis muscle
- help from below
- rotation to OA

Uterus
- high enough incision into the lower segment
- use of bandage scissors
- smile-shaped uterotomy
- avoid MROP
- swift identification of angles and haemostatic sutures, exteriorisation of the uterus may be neccessary

The essay itself

A second-stage Caesarean section after failed instrumental delivery is a potentially difficult procedure. The woman is positioned supine on the table with a slight, left-lateral tilt. The difficulties of this operation may arise from a high riding bladder and a deeply impacted fetal head. To keep the bladder empty, an indwelling Foley's catheter should be inserted before starting the procedure. Haemorrhage, infection and thromboembolism are also of concern.

A large enough skin incision, the rectus sheath and separation of the pyramidalis muscle (if present) should be performed to create enough space.

In some cases an extra person is required to push the deeply impacted fetal head up, thereby facilitating delivery.

Haemorrhage may occur from the uterus or the vagina. A high enough incision should be performed into the lower segment, avoiding cervical and vaginal tissues. A smile-shaped uterotomy is done and manually extended to guide potential tears upwards into the uterus rather than the broad ligament. Rotation of the head to the occipitoanterior position not only eases delivery but also prevents tears into the broad ligament and vagina. The placenta should be delivered by controlled cord traction rather than manual removal, and the uterine cavity emptied of any residual placental tissue. A contraction can be rubbed up by the assistant while the surgeon swiftly identifies and secures the angles of the uterotomy. The uterus may need to be extraterritorised to identify the full length of the incision and also to repair broad ligament tears. A double-layer closure of the uterotomy would be justified for haemostatic purposes. Additional bleeding points should be temporarily secured with Green Armitages before haemostatic sutures, eg figures of eight sutures are preferable to diathermy. Hysterectomy should be anticipated and not delayed if haemorrhage cannot be controlled. A Sim's speculum examination should be performed at the end to identify and repair any trauma to the lower birth canal.

High upward preparation of the rectus sheath, identification of the visceral peritoneum and careful opening of the same can prevent bladder injuries. The bladder should be protected at all times with the Doyen's retractor. Methylene blue can be injected into the bladder via the Foley's catheter and tears localised and repaired.

Clear documentation is vitally important.

Essay 25

A 33-year-old woman has had two second trimester losses in the past. She is now 13 weeks' pregnant and requests cervical cerclage.

Would you support her request?

Essay tips
The key words in this question are:

- all of the first sentence
- 13 weeks' pregnant – requests cerclage
- would you support her request

The first sentence
Obviously your level of suspicion would be high enough by now to question whether this was the full story. Therefore you first take a history. Areas of interest would be any other pregnancy outcome, eg:

- first trimester loss (termination of pregnancy (TOP), miscarriage)
- preterm labour
- term deliveries.

Specific to these second trimester losses you need to know:

- whether they were painless
- preceded by premature rupture of membranes
- whether any investigation results are available such as:
  - parenteral and fetal karyotyping
  - maternal thrombophilia screen
  - known uterine abnormality
  - vaginal swab results.

She may have had a previous cerclage, which had failed. Does she have any connective tissue disorder?

13 weeks' pregnant – requests cerclage
Here the dilemma starts, and this is exactly the area the College wants you to deal with. You need to consider the following points:

- Cerclage is the treatment for cervical incompetence.

- However, cervical incompetence, as such, is a diagnosis of exclusion without its own definition. One way of finding out is from the woman's past obstetric history.
- Aside from the fact that history alone is not very reliable, a clinical diagnosis of cervical incompetence in a previous pregnancy does not necessarily indicate there would be any benefit from a cervical suture in the present pregnancy.
- Statistically, 25 cerclages have to be performed to prevent one preterm birth.

But here she wants her suture.

- Clearly her risk of a preterm birth with two second trimester losses is significantly increased, regardless of whether her cervix was ever competent or not.
- The procedure-related risk of pregnancy loss together with that of general anaesthesia is certainly smaller than the risk of a recurrent preterm birth.
- She may also be happy enough to tolerate some discharge throughout her pregnancy and a higher risk of puerperal pyrexia and medical intervention.

Would you support her request?

Needless to say, this is not a 'yes' or 'no' question.

Are there any alternatives?

- Well, she could be offered transvaginal scans at regular intervals. However, if she truly had cervical incompetence her cervix may dilate at any time without warning. Even if there was time, the expected result of a rescue suture is rather poor.
- Vaginal pessaries (eg Smith–Hodge pessaries) have performed well in the MRC/RCOG trial and could be offered instead of surgery and anaesthesia.
- If you were to offer a cervical cerclage, the MacDonald procedure is the easier option compared to Shirodkar since no bladder dissection is needed. The success rate is roughly the same.
- Transabdominal cerclage claims a success rate of 85–93% but is obviously more invasive. However, if this woman has no living children and had previously failed vaginal approaches – as you may find out in the history – the above may be an option. Elective Caesarean section would then be the mode of delivery.

The essay itself

Careful counselling of this woman and her partner is necessary to reach a sensible decision.

History

A comprehensive history needs to be taken first, including details of other pregnancy outcomes, eg first trimester losses (termination of pregnancy or miscarriage), preterm labours and term deliveries. Painless pregnancy losses preceded by premature rupture of membranes would support the diagnosis of cervical incompetence. Her notes should be reviewed and other results of investigations enquired into, such as parenteral and fetal karyotyping, a maternal thrombophilia screen and vaginal swab results and postmortem reports. She may have a known uterine anomaly or connective tissue disorder necessitating different treatment options.

Counselling

History-taking should be followed by a balanced discussion of the potential benefits and drawbacks of cervical cerclage and include possible alternatives. It should be highlighted that cerclage is the treatment for cervical incompetence but that its diagnosis is one of exclusion. A clinical diagnosis of cervical incompetence in a previous pregnancy does not necessarily indicate any benefits from a cervical suture in the present pregnancy. Overall, 25 cerclages need to be performed to prevent one preterm birth. On the other hand, this woman's risk of a preterm birth with two second trimester losses is certainly significantly increased regardless of whether her cervix was ever competent or not. It is also worthwhile to mention that the procedure-related risk of pregnancy loss together with the added risk of regional anaesthesia is relatively small. Cerclage may cause more vaginal discharge throughout pregnancy and a higher risk of puerperal pyrexia and medical intervention.

If a cervical cerclage was offered, the MacDonald's' suture is somewhat easier to perform then a Shirodkar suture since no bladder dissection is necessary. The success rates are similar.

Transabdominal cerclage has a success rate of 85–93%, but is obviously more invasive since it involves a laparotomy. Delivery would be by elective Caesarean section. However, if this woman has no living children and/or a previously failed vaginal approach transabdominal cerclage may still be an option.

As an alternative, transvaginal scanning could be offered to assess the cervical length and also to look out for features like funneling and beaking. The procedure has the advantage of being minimally invasive and can be repeated at any time. However, if this woman truly had cervical incompetence her cervix could dilate at any time without warning, and even if there was time for a rescue suture the result of this would be expected to be rather poor.

Non-surgical alternatives would be vaginal pessaries, eg the Smith–Hodge pessary or even a shelf pessary, the former having a proven infant survival rate of 91% versus 22% with expectant management. The MRCOG/RCOG trial has also shown an improved neonatal outcome in terms of delivery after both 33 and 37 weeks' gestation.

Throughout the counselling session the couple's views and aspirations need to be taken into consideration at all times.

OSCES

Station 1

Candidate instructions

Mr and Mrs Smith have been referred to you for counselling after Mrs Smith's 12-week ultrasound scan.

12-week scan report:

Monochorionic diamniotic twin pregnancy

Fetus 1 – CRL 75 mm, fetal heart beat seen, nuchal translucency (NT) 22 mm

Fetus 2 – CRL 77 mm, fetal heart beat seen, nuchal translucency (NT) 34 mm.

- Age-related risk of Down's syndrome 1:652
- Fetus 2 adjusted risk of Down's syndrome 1:123

Discuss with the examiner the specific counselling you would give Mr and Mrs Smith, and why.

Examiner's mark sheet

1 Candidate explains the need to know more about Mrs Smith's obstetric history (parity, previous aneuploidy, age, fertility and if this was a planned pregnancy). **1 mark**

2 Explains what nuchal translucency is, counsels sensitively, keeps medical jargon to a minimum and gives facts and information, candidate says they would not make the decision for Mrs Smith – it is her choice. Reiterates that only when Mrs Smith has been fully informed of the options and risks can she make a decision – the decision is hers, not the doctor's. **1 mark**

3 Explains that although NT T1 is normal, T2 is abnormally high, and therefore invasive testing would be offered. **1 mark**

4 Explains that invasive testing is an option but is not mandatory. **1 mark**

5 Explains the option of biochemical screening (second trimester) in addition to the above, and says that it may give a different risk value. **1 mark**

6 Explains that both chorionic villous sampling (CVS) and amniocentesis are performed with a single-pass needle, and are used to determine the karyotype of both twins. **1 mark**

7 Explains the advantages and disadvantages of CVS versus amniocentesis:

- Advantages:
  - mainly the early result (Fluorescence *In-Situ* Hybridisation (FISH) 48 h; full culture results in 7–14 days).

- Disadvantages:
  - failure to culture
  - mosaicism
  - increased risk of miscarriage. **1 mark**

8 Explains that even if the chromosome analysis is normal, there is still a small risk of cardiac abnormalities and other rare genetic syndromes. **1 mark**

9 Explains the need for further scans because of the risks associated with monochorionic twin pregnancies, including: preterm delivery, twin–twin transfusion syndrome and intrauterine growth retardation (IUGR). **2 marks**

Station 2

Candidate instructions

Mr and Mrs Williams have come for the results of Mrs Williams's 20-week ultrasound scan.

20-week anomaly ultrasound scan report:

Mild ventriculomegaly, lumbosacral meningocoele evident

Bilateral talipes

Liquor volume normal, fetal anatomy and biometry consistent with dates.

Explain the significance of the ultrasound scan report to the examiner and say how you would counsel/advise the patient.

Examiner's mark sheet

1 Explains that a meningocoele is an open neural tube defect and that it does not contain neural tissue unlike a meningomyelocoele, so the former has a better prognosis. **1 mark**

2 Explains that the lumbosacral region is the most common site; and that the lower the lesion, the better the prognosis. **1 mark**

3 Explains that ventriculomegaly is often associated with lumbosacral spina bifida and can be associated with aneuploidy (consider amniocentesis), other central nervous system defects and congenital infections. **1 mark**

4 Explains that talipes is often associated with lumbosacral spina bifida and may respond to physiotherapy or surgery. **1 mark**

5 Explains that an affected child may have voiding difficulties in the long term. **1 mark**

6 Explains that the mother would be asked about her medical history, including whether she has ever had epilepsy, used periconceptual folic acid or had a previous pregnancy with a neural tube defect. **1 mark**

7 The candidate would tell the parents they have the option to see a paediatrician/neurosurgeon to discuss the prognosis. **1 mark**

8 Says the option of terminating or continuing the pregnancy would be discussed with the parent(s). **1 mark**

9 Explains that the mode of delivery would be discussed with the parents – Caesarean section versus vaginal delivery – a lower segment Caesarean section would be offered, but the optimal route is debatable. **1 mark**

10 Discusses increasing the dose of folate for future pregnancies, and requesting possible 16-week α-fetoprotein/ultrasound screening. **1 mark**

Station 3

Candidate instructions

In this role-play, you are required to take a relevant history from Mrs Jones who has been referred to you by the day assessment-unit midwife with a blood pressure reading of 160/115 and 1+ proteinuria.

Indicate to the examiner the appropriate investigations you may want to request (and why) and discuss possible treatment options with this 'patient'.

Role player's instructions

- You are 37 years of age and in your second pregnancy.
- Your first pregnancy was seven years ago and resulted in a male infant delivered at 40 weeks by Caesarean section for failure to progress at 7-cm dilatation after being induced for pre-eclampsia.
- You are now 39 weeks' pregnant.
- This was an unplanned pregnancy and you are planning to give the child up for adoption after its birth.
- You are separated from your husband and this pregnancy is by another man.
- You have had a persistent frontal headache for the last 12 hours that is not settling.
- You are currently unemployed, do not smoke, take drugs or drink alcohol.
- You have had no problems in the pregnancy until now.
- You are otherwise fit and well and have had no other operations or medical conditions of note, you take no medication and are not allergic to anything.
- The midwife has palpated your abdomen and, although baby is 'head down', she feels that you are small for dates.
- Ask the candidate if you can go home as you are keen to get back to your son.
- Ask the candidate if you and the baby will be alright.
- If possible, say you would like to avoid a Caesarean section this time.

Examiner's mark sheet

1 The candidate makes good eye contact, has good rapport, listens to the patient appropriately. **1 mark**

2 Discusses the risks for pre-eclampsia (previous pre-eclampsia, different partner, age). **1 mark**

3 Takes a general history. **1 mark**

4 Requests appropriate investigations: mid-stream urine sample for culture; 24-hour urine collection for protein estimation; FBC; urea and electrolytes, including urate; liver function tests; and clotting times. **2 marks**

5 Shows an appreciation of the pros and cons of treatment (antihypertensives/wait to see if BP settles). **1 mark**

6 Is aware that induction of labour may be an option if the cervix is favourable, and is aware of the small (2.5%) risk of scar rupture from the previous Caesarean section. The candidate has considered using the Bishop's score and artificial rupture of membranes instead of prostaglandin induction of labour. **2 marks**

7 Discusses the option and pros/cons of a semi-elective/non-urgent Caesarean section. **2 marks**

Station 4

Candidate instructions

Miss Peak, 23 years of age, has been referred to you by her GP with amenorrhoea for six months and galactorrhoea of three months' duration. Her serum prolactin level is 7600 IU.

Explain to the examiner those specific relevant features you would want to elicit from her history, the relevant investigations you may require and how you may manage her.

Examiner's mark sheet

1 History:
   - candidate appreciates this patient could be pregnant, have recently been pregnant, have finished breast-feeding
   - on medication causing galactorrhoea
   - has visual impairment
   - has symptoms of thyroid disease
   - has a previous history of similar problems.

   2 marks

2 Investigations:
   - would request a pregnancy test
   - serum prolactin assay (split assay/active/inactive)
   - thyroid function tests
   - FSH/LH assays
   - ultrasound scan of the pelvis
   - MRI/CT scan of the pituitary fossa.

   3 marks

3 Treatment:

   Examiner to say that all investigations are normal, except for a raised prolactin level and a pituitary adenoma. The examiner to ask the candidate how s(he) would treat the patient.

   - Carefully and simply explains the treatment options to the patient.
     - Would await the results of the pituitary scan, then:
     - if prolactin > 8000 IU and prolactinoma < 1 cm would treat with drugs (bromocriptine versus cabergoline)
     - if prolactin < 3000 IU and prolactinoma > 1 cm says that surgical referral may be more appropriate.

   3 marks

4 **Examiner asks the candidate how s(he) would manage the patient if she is pregnant.**

Candidate says that the prolactin level is difficult to monitor as it is raised in pregnancy, but the patient would need pituitary fossa imaging if her visual symptoms or headaches persist. Explains that bromocriptine can be safely given and the mother can breast-feed; says there is no need to alter the mode of delivery.

2 marks

Station 5

Candidate instructions

Explain to the examiner how you would manage a case of postpartum haemorrhage. The examiner prompts you that the patient is still bleeding after each suggestion you make.

Examiner's mark sheet

1 Candidate would assess the patient's airway, breathing, circulation; site large-bore intravenous cannulas; take blood for a full blood count, clotting, cross-match (initially 4–6 units). Give blood (and fresh-frozen plasma with every 6 units, and consider giving cryoprecipitate if the patient has a very low fibrinogen level), maintain a strict fluid-balance chart, central line and urinary catheter. As appropriate, would explain the situation to the patient and her partner, inform them of what steps s(he) is taking and why. **2 marks**

2 The candidate would look for causes of the haemorrhage, and explains that in most cases this will be an atonic uterus; says they would evacuate clots, remove retained products/placenta if necessary and examine for cervical or vaginal tears. **1 mark**

3 Would make sure the uterus is well contracted: manually rub up a contraction/apply bimanual pressure; give 5 IU oxytocin as an i.v. bolus and ergometrine 0.5 mg. **1mark**

4 Would give carboprost intramuscularly, 250 μg every 15 minutes up to a maximum of eight doses. Candidate explains that if the patient loses > 1.5 litres of blood, the consultant obstetrician should be informed as well as the duty consultant haematologist and anaesthetist. **1 mark**

5 Would consider packing the uterus with gauze or gauze soaked in prostaglandin gel, misoprostol pessaries or intramyometral carboprost. **1mark**

6 Explains that a balloon tamponade using an intrauterine balloon catheter and vaginal pack may be highly effective. **1mark**

7 Would consider radiological embolisation of the uterine arteries with a gelatin sponge. **1 mark**

8 Would consider a B-Lynch suture (if due to uterine atony), or ligation of uterine arteries, or anterior division of the internal iliac arteries. Explains that using a bulldog clip first can assess the effectiveness of each. **1 mark**

9 Would consider a subtotal hysterectomy with ovarian conservation if bleeding persists or haemorrhage becomes uncontrollable. **1 mark**

Station 6

Candidate instructions

Ms Duke is 38 years of age, nulliparous, HIV-positive with large bilateral hydrosalpinges. She, together with her female partner, wishes to have a baby in the very near future and wants to ask you some questions. Counsel her appropriately.

Examiner's mark sheet

How can I become pregnant?

1 Advises *in-vitro* fertilisation (IVF) with donor sperm.

2 Says that, although salpingostomy and donor intrauterine insemination (IUI) is possible, it is not recommended in women with severe tubal disease. **2 marks**

Can I get assisted conception/IVF through the National Health Service?

1 Advises her that her age needs to be considered:

- The recent NICE guideline recommends IVF on the NHS for women under 40 years of age.

2 Explains that the severity of her HIV disease needs to be considered:

- What is her CD4 count?
- Does she have any AIDS-like illnesses?
- What is her viral load and is she on antiretroviral agents (these can affect embryogenesis)? Says a report from her HIV physicians will be needed.

3 Advises that her partner's HIV status also needs consideration:

- Tells her that the local infertility ethics committee (the IVF co-ordinator, holder of HFEA (Human Fertilization and Embryology Authority) licence, embryologist, counsellor and genitourinary medicine physicians) will need to be involved.
- Advises her of the need to consider the welfare of her unborn child – HIV transmission.
- Explains that she will need to give details of her general history, any convictions, any psychiatric history and her hepatitis B and C status.
- Says that information (demographics, etc) on her partner will also be needed.
- Explains that, although lesbian status is not a contraindication, it will need to be discussed by the ethics committee and can involve HFEA guidance. **3 marks**

If I am granted IVF on the NHS, are there any specific precautions you would take in view of my HIV status and bilateral hydrosalpinges?

1 Candidate says they would advise tubal ligation as this gives a better implantation rate.

2 Involve the GU-medicine unit to monitor Ms Duke's CD4 count, viral load and disease progression.

3 Use non-maternal plasma culture medium for the embryos and culture them in a separate incubator to non-HIV embryos.

4 Advise that if pregnancy is achieved, she will need antiretroviral therapy during pregnancy and an elective Caesarean section; and will need to bottle-feed to reduce the risk of vertical transmission to the baby.

5 Perform a PCR test on infant blood to exclude the vertical transmission of HIV. **2 marks**

Would it also be possible for me to have donor eggs from a younger/HIV-negative woman – I would be willing to pay her for them?

1 Advises her that:

- It is illegal to pay for eggs in the UK (only expenses are allowed).
- There is usually a waiting list as few eggs are donated in the UK. **1 mark**

I have a male friend who is HIV-positive and I would like him to be the sperm donor, is this possible? We would also like to have a girl – I gather the sperm can be separated to make this possible? Alternatively, could we have a preimplantation diagnosis to check that it is a girl?

1 Advises her that:

- More information about the male donor would be needed – his CD4 count, general and psychiatric history, etc; as well as discussion by the local ethics committee and HFEA advice. In general, provided the donor is suitable after an ethics committee review and HFEA guidelines are followed then sperm washing may be undertaken.

- Sex selection for non-sex-linked conditions is illegal in the UK.

- Preimplantation diagnosis cannot be undertaken for social reasons in the UK, and this could significantly reduce the implantation/pregnancy rates. **1 mark**

What is involved in IVF and what are the risks?

1 Explains: natural/short/long-cycle regimens; superovulation with gonadotrophins; follicle tracking; time off work; the success rate of around 15%, depending on her age and the unit; the risks of ovarian hyperstimulation syndrome; ovarian accidents; multiple pregnancy; vertical transmission risk and the long-term risk of ovarian cancer with superovulation. **1 mark**

Station 7

Candidate instructions

Mrs Jones is 31 years of age and in her first pregnancy. She attended the booking clinic at 16 weeks' gestation and is now 18 weeks pregnant. She is referred to you with the results of her booking blood test for rubella, and for a history of malaise, flu-like symptoms and a pinpoint macular rash that appeared two days ago. She did not receive rubella vaccination at school.

Microbiology laboratory report

HIA rubella IgG = < 10 (non-immune)

HIA/MAC-RIA rubella IgM = positive.

She would like to know the significance of the test result, the implications for her pregnancy and what her options are for this pregnancy.

Examiner's mark sheet

1 The candidate gives a simple explanation of what rubella is (a virus) and what the test results mean; says it is unlikely they are the result of past exposure to rubella, but are likely to be due to a recent exposure. **2 marks**

2 Explains where the infection may have come from (contact), and the need to stay away from pregnant women for 8 days after the onset of the rubella rash. **1 mark**

3 Explains that, although she has recently had rubella, it does not mean that her baby will invariably be infected or affected by it. Explains the risks of congenital infection if exposure occurs at 16 weeks' gestation (infection rate in fetuses is approximately 50% and congenital defects are present in about 50% of these). **1 mark**

4 Explains that the rash usually occurs about 16 days after exposure to the rubella virus, so she was probably exposed to the virus at around 16 weeks' gestation. **1 mark**

5 Explains the need for follow-up in the fetal medicine centre or with a consultant virologist to discuss possible further investigations, including cordocentesis (to establish if the fetus is infected). Explains that the risk of miscarriage with such a procedure is approximately 2%. **2 marks**

6 Explains that a termination of pregnancy is an option, and briefly describes how this is done. The candidate suggests referral to another practitioner if she has a moral objection to termination. Explains that she does not need to be vaccinated as she will now have natural immunity. **1 mark**

7 Explains that abnormalities may not be seen on ultrasound (deafness, retinopathy, cataracts, mental retardation, hepatosplenomegaly, Diabetes Mellitus in the child's twenties, meningitis, hypotonia) – although IUGR may be present, as may pulmonary valvular stenosis and patent ductus arteriosus.

Explains that she can be referred to the paediatrician to discuss the longer term prognosis. **1 mark**

8 Explains that in the worst-case scenario of congenital infection, the baby may die *in utero*. Alternatively, it could be born with a handicap, in which case she could see a paediatrician to discuss the longer term prognosis. **1 mark**

Station 8

Candidate instructions

You are performing a total abdominal hysterectomy with ovarian conservation and you want to use diathermy for haemostasis. However, in spite of sustained pressure on the diathermy pedal nothing happens. Explain what actions you would take, and discuss the use of diathermy with the examiner.

Examiner's mark sheet

1 Candidate explains they would first check that the machine was switched on, that the diathermy unit was properly connected to the machine and to the patient pad (if monopolar). The candidate would check that the output settings were high enough to produce an effect and consider changing the lead if the problem persisted. Says they would ensure they were pressing on the diathermy pedal rather than on the cutting pedal. **1 mark**

2 Explains the differences between monopolar and bipolar settings:
   • Monopolar means the current passes through the patient's body, and may result in a larger dissipation of heat energy compared to bipolar diathermy where the current acts between the two local electrodes. **2 marks**

3 Explains the different forms of monopolar coagulation:
   • Spray – delivers superficial, high voltage, is not in contact with tissue, and is good for use under water or for a diffused haemorrhage.
   • Fulguration – delivers high voltage with a good depth of coagulation to major bleeds.
   • Desiccation – produces a slow drying out of tissues with the electrode in contact with tissues; it is the most commonly used. **1 mark**

4 Explains which modality they would use to cut through:
   • the skin – monopolar cutting diathermy with blend; for cutting and haemostasis without the need for a precise limit of heat damage to tissue
   • the rectus sheath – monopolar cutting diathermy with blend; for cutting and haemostasis without the need for a precise limit of heat damage to tissue
   • to obtain haemostasis at the ovarian pedicle – bipolar diathermy; to obtain precise haemostasis and to limit heat damage to the surrounding tissues, eg to the ureter. **2 marks**

5 Explains which settings they would set the machine to. Says the exact value is unimportant, but a reasonable setting would be 35 diathermy and 35 cutting with blend. **1 mark**

6 Explains what they would do if they noticed a burning smell after closing the skin at the end of the procedure:
   - Candidate would check the leg pad on the patient for skin burns – check if it was properly applied flush to the skin or not. If a skin burn was noticed, the candidate would fill out a risk-management form, inform the head theatre sister and consultant in charge of the case, ask the advice of a plastic surgeon and explain the incident to the patient. **2 marks**

7 Explains how the chances of injury could be minimised when using diathermy in gynaecological surgery.
   - Put the electrode in its holster in between use – do not leave the electrodes on the patient.
   - Do not use high-voltage spray coagulation.
   - Use low-voltage desiccation coagulation.
   - Be aware of a direct coupling risk.
   - Use a bipolar technique if possible.
   - Always check the integrity of instruments/cable insulation of electrodes.
   - Follow audit department guidelines on the use of diathermy.
   - Discuss relevant issues with the departmental risk manager.
   - Ensure risk management forms/trigger response forms are filled out appropriately. **1 mark**

Station 9

Candidate instructions

You are asked to advise this young 18-year-old woman about her contraceptive options. Explain your advice to her.

Examiner's mark list

1 The candidate says they would ask the patient if she really requires contraception at this point; ask if she is in a relationship; ask when she had her last menstrual period; and ask if she has any salient medical conditions that may alter the advice given. **2 marks**

2 Explains the different types of temporary contraception:
- hormonal – oral contraceptive pill, depo injection, implant, Mirena coil
- barrier methods – condom, cap, diaphragm
- intra-uterine devices – copper and inert devices. **2 marks**

3 Explains the permanent methods of contraception, including sterilisation; explains this is not routinely recommended for such young women. **2 marks**

4 Advises 'Double Dutch' contraception (ie protection from infections such as chlamydia by using condoms, and also a reliable contraceptive method such as the pill or the depo injection). **2 marks**

5 Asks her if she has any particular preferences. **2 marks**

6 The candidate explains how they would advise her if she wishes to try the combined oral contraceptive pill – and advise on how she should take it:
- Informs her that she starts taking the pill at the beginning of her period and continues to take it up to day 21 of her cycle, then she stops and has a withdrawal bleed for 7 or less days. Explains that contraception is effective immediately if taken from day 1 of her cycle.
- Explains what to do if is late taking a pill (> 12 hours) – take the next pill as soon as possible and use barrier methods for the next 7 days. If the missed pill is at the end of the packet (after day 14) then continue onto the next packet of pills without a break. Explains to her to do the same if she is prescribed antibiotics or has diarrhoea or vomiting as both situations may impair absorption of the pill. **2 marks**

7 Explains the side-effects of the combined oral contraceptive pill:

- Explains the risk of thromboembolic disease. Says they would not prescribe it to women who have a personal or family history of congenital or acquired thrombophilia, to heavy smokers, over 35, with cardiovascular disease, high blood pressure or women with uncontrolled diabetes or diabetes with micro/macrovascular disease. Explains that a woman who is taking enzyme-inducing drugs may need a higher dose of the pill. **2 marks**

8 Explains when the patient should seek emergency contraception:

- If unprotected sexual intercourse occurred or she missed two or more pills in the first seven days or the last seven days of a packet (if a new packet was not started immediately and she had a seven-day break).
- If four or more pills (in any combination) were missed mid-packet.
- 1 day on antibiotics = 1 day missed pill. **2 marks**

9 Explains the different forms of emergency contraception:

- Currently licensed options are the combined estrogen and progesterone pill, and the progesterone-only pill (two doses of 0.75 mg levonorgestrel 12 hours apart; however, if vomiting occurs within 3 hours then another tablet has to be taken).
- Explains that the progesterone-only method is more effective and has less side-effects than PC4, although both can be taken up to 72 hours after unprotected sexual intercourse.
- If unprotected sexual intercourse occurred more than 72 hours but less than 5 days ago, she can use the copper coil (failure rate 0.4–2.4 per 100 woman-years).
- Explains the need for follow-up to check that her next period is not late and to screen for sexually transmitted diseases if necessary. Explains the coil would be removed with her next period if required. **2 marks**

Station 10

Candidate instructions

A 20-year-old pregnant, insulin-dependent diabetic woman attends for her very first antenatal booking visit at 22 weeks' gestation. Explain how you would counsel her.

Examiner's mark sheet

1 Asks: if she has any other relevant history; other medical illnesses; takes other medications; if this is her first pregnancy or not; how long she has been diabetic for and what is her level of diabetic control; and if she has had any scans to confirm her dates. **1 mark**

2 Explains that booking normally occurs earlier than 22 weeks. However, the candidate reassures her and explains the need to arrange various appointments. **1 mark**

3 Candidate says they would arrange a multidisciplinary (obstetrician or physician with an interest in obstetric medicine, diabetic nurse specialist, midwife, dietician) clinic appointment to closely monitor blood-glucose control (aim for preprandial levels < 6 and postprandial levels < 8 mmol/l – via home blood-glucose monitoring). Explains that good blood-glucose control will help the health of both the mother and the baby. **1 mark**

4 Candidate would arrange booking blood tests (full blood count, blood group and antibody check, syphilis serology, hepatitis B serology, HIV serology (with consent), renal function and glycosylated haemoglobin (Hb Alc) (for average blood sugars over the last 6–8 weeks). Obtain a mid-stream urine sample for microscopy, culture and sensitivity (as asymptomatic bacteriuria may be present) and bedside testing for microalbuminuria, suggestive of renal impairment. **1 mark**

5 Would explain the need for an ultrasound scan if she has not had one. Explains that this will estimate the gestational age (especially if she is uncertain of the date of her last menstrual period or her periods had been irregular); will check for congenital anomalies, number of fetuses and location of the placenta. This is important because babies born to diabetic women have a higher risk of congenital anomalies than those born to non-diabetic women. **1 mark**

6 Explains that it may be more difficult to screen for chromosomal anomalies at this gestation (too late for nuchal translucency and

is at the maximum limit for serum biochemical screening). The candidate would counsel that 'soft markers' on ultrasound may help to screen for chromosomal abnormalities, although they are not very sensitive or specific unless two or more are present. Explains that she could have cordocentesis, although the risk of miscarriage would be at least 2%. **1 mark**

5 Explains the need for hospital-based and consultant-led care throughout the pregnancy (as she is in a higher risk group). **1 mark**

6 The candidate would arrange further tests for Hb Alc, and serial scans to monitor fetal growth and amniotic fluid volume at around 28, 32 and 36 weeks' gestation (diabetic babies may be macrosomic or have polyhydramnios or even exhibit IUGR). **1 mark**

7 Explains the risks of diabetic pregnancy: poor blood-sugar control/hypoglycaemia, retinopathy and renal dysfunction, macrosomia, shoulder dystocia, infections, preterm labour, high blood pressure, congenital anomalies, neonatal respiratory-distress syndrome, neonatal hypoglycaemia, neonatal admission in the immediate postpartum period and the small increased risk of intrauterine death. Would reassure her that with close monitoring and appropriate management most diabetic pregnancies do not experience such complications. **1 mark**

8 Counsels her that she may consider induction of labour at 38–39 weeks' gestation (to avoid the risk of intrauterine death). **1 mark**

9 Explains that her insulin requirement is likely to increase, especially during the last trimester, and that postnatally this will return to her prepregnant levels. **1 mark**

10 Asks her if she has any questions or needs clarification of any of the points raised. **1 mark**

Station 11

Candidate instructions

A woman presents to you in the antenatal clinic at 17 weeks' gestation with an ultrasound scan report showing an increased nuchal fat pad of 45 mm in the fetus and no other anomalies. This is her first ultrasound scan. Explain how you would counsel her.

Examiner's mark sheet

1 Candidate explains the need to obtain a medical history from her, including whether this is her first pregnancy and if not, any history of this in previous pregnancies and whether she knows of any genetic/chromosomal problems in the family. Has she had serum biochemical screening yet? Is there any history of viral infections in this pregnancy? **1 mark**

2 Explains what the ultrasound scan has shown – an increased area of thickness in the soft tissue between the skin and the spine at the back of the baby's neck. Also reiterates that no other abnormalities have been seen. **1 mark**

3 Explains that most women have this scan between 11 and 14 weeks and that the fluid behind the neck at this time is called 'nuchal translucency' (which all fetuses have to some degree and which disappears by 14 weeks in most cases). After 14 weeks' gestation, the presence of a sonolucent area may represent extra fluid that may be slowly resolving (nuchal translucency) or be a sign of hydrops (fetal heart failure) or it may be an extra area of tissue that is a variant of normal. **1 mark**

4 Explains that such a finding may be associated with chromosomal abnormalities like Down's syndrome or heart anomalies. In the absence of other markers, this is unlikely. (Unless you are certain of your figures do not give a specific risk figure of the likelihood of chromosomal abnormality.) Explains that she would be referred to the local fetal medicine unit for risk assessment and possibly fetal echocardiography. **1 mark**

5 Explains that such a finding may be a normal variant and there is every chance the baby will be normal, although this cannot be guaranteed. Explains that one option would be to wait until the 20-week scan to check all the baby's anatomy, although most fetal medicine units should be able to see most anomalies by now. Moreover, if she opted for a termination, the earlier this was done, the safer for her. **1 mark**

6 Explains that the only way to exclude a chromosomal abnormality would be by invasive testing (such as amniocentesis). Explains that this involves passing a small needle through the mother's abdomen to obtain some fluid from the baby. Explain that initial results may be available in 3–5 days, and the full culture results in 10–14 days. Explains there is a small risk of failed culture and a 1% risk of miscarriage with such a procedure. **1 mark**

7 Counsels her that the risks of having an affected child need to be weighed against the risks of miscarriage, and that the fetal medicine unit is best qualified to give her the exact risks involved. **1 mark**

8 Explains that the neck thickness may become greater as the pregnancy progresses, but that it usually regresses and is unlikely to be evident at birth. **1 mark**

9 Explains that if she wanted to terminate the pregnancy this could be arranged, although the candidate would advise going to the fetal-medicine unit first. Candidate would only explain the methods of termination if she asks for this information.
1 mark

10 Asks if she has any further questions she would like answered.

Station 12

Candidate instructions

On the morning you are due to perform a total abdominal hysterectomy with ovarian conservation, your patient says that she now wishes to have a subtotal hysterectomy and bilateral salpingo-oophorectomy (BSO). Explain your counselling and actions. The examiner may ask you to describe the operative procedure of total or subtotal abdominal hysterectomy and oophorectomy.

Examiner's mark sheet

1 The candidate would ask the patient if she is sure this is what she wants and asks why she has changed her mind. **1 mark**

2 Explains the pros and cons of total versus subtotal hysterectomy:
   * Pros:
     – Removal of the cervix, so there is no need for further smears (providing histology and previous smears were normal).
     – There is also a lesser risk (negligible risk) of vaginal spotting/bleeding than after a subtotal hysterectomy.

   * Cons:
     – Removal of the cervix will require further dissection of the bladder and the operation may take longer.
     – The previous belief that total hysterectomy led to increased risks of voiding, sexual and bowel disorders has not been supported by recent randomised controlled trials. The subject is, however, still controversial. **1 mark**

3 Explains the pros and cons of bilateral salpingo-oophorectomy and conservation:
   * Pros:
     – Removing the ovaries and tubes removes the background risk of developing ovarian carcinoma (approximately 1 in 70 lifetime risk if no family history) or fallopian tube cancer (extremely rare anyway).
     – It also removes her risk of developing benign ovarian cysts in later life.

   * Cons:
     – Removing the ovaries in the vast majority of women of reproductive age will result in the acute onset of menopausal symptoms, including hot flushes, sweats, mood swings, tiredness and vaginal dryness within the first postoperative week. This may necessitate the need for hormone-replacement therapy, the pros and cons of which also need to be explained to the patient.
     – Reassures the patient that there is no real disadvantage in removing the fallopian tubes. **2 marks**

4 Explains the pros and cons of using HRT:

- Pros:
  - Improves mood swings, hot sweats, dry vagina, libido, skin, teeth, muscular aches/pains.
  - Reduces the risk of osteoporosis and colon cancer.

- Cons:
  - There is an increased risk of deep-vein thrombosis (DVT) from 10:100 000 to 30 in 100 000, and an increased risk of breast cancer from 45/1000 to 90 in 1000 over an 8-year period of use.
  - Explains that increased risks of stroke and ischaemic heart disease have been associated with HRT, but chiefly with the combined oestrogen and progestagen type (which will not be applicable to her if she had a hysterectomy). **2 marks**

5 Explains that after careful counselling, if the patient was absolutely happy with her new decision, had no further questions and was willing to sign a new updated consent form, then the candidate would be happy to go ahead with a subtotal hysterectomy with BSO this morning. Should there be any doubt in the patient's mind, then the operation would be cancelled to allow her more time to consider her options.

2 marks

6 Explains [if the examiner asks] how a subtotal abdominal hysterectomy with BSO would be performed.

- Takes the examiner through each preparatory step:
  - positioning the patient on the operating table
  - performing a vaginal examination to ascertain the size and mobility of the uterus
  - catheterisation (in-dwelling or single-pass silver catheter)
  - use of methylene blue or not
  - what solution would be used to clean the skin (iodine or chlorhexidine), how the sterile drapes would be placed and discusses the use of prophylactic antibiotics perioperatively.

- Then describes the procedure:
  - Make a lower transverse incision (if the uterus is not too big).

- Make a careful knife dissection through the skin and complete the rest of the dissection through the fat/muscle rectus sheath–diathermy blade to minimise blood loss.
- Use Mayo scissors to cut through the rectus sheath.
- Divide the rectus muscles in the mid-line.
- Enter the peritoneum using Spencer–Wells forceps to pull the parietal peritoneum away from the underlying bowel and incise it with the scalpel.
- Carefully extend the incision by gently stretching the peritoneum.
- Carefully place a self-retaining retractor and use wet packs to hold back the intestines from the operative field.
- Place two Kocher's forceps adjacent to the uterus on the left and right sides. Some operators prefer Spencer-Wells as they are less traumatic.
- Put a Spencer–Wells forceps on the round ligament on one side and cut through with the curved Mayo scissors; tie with Vicryl, and open up the broad ligament anteriorly and posteriorly. Identify the ovarian vessels at the pelvic brim and put a finger through the remaining leaf of broad ligament to isolate the ovarian pedicle, then place a curved Gwillim clamp over the ovarian pedicle with a Spencer–Wells to prevent back flow of blood. Some operators would suggest you identify the ureter prior to this procedure. Divide the infundibulopelvic ligament between the clamps and double tie the pedicle with 1 Vicryl. Repeat the process on the other side.
- Using the curved Mayo scissors, carefully open the uterovesical peritoneum from right to left and carefully reflect the bladder down with a small swab in the mid-line. Check that the ureters are below and lateral to the uterine artery.
- Place a Gwillim clamp over the uterine pedicle with a Spencer–Wells to prevent backflow, then cut between the clamps and double tie the uterine artery pedicle with 1 Vicryl.
- Ensuring the bladder is well reflected from the cervix, put a swab behind the cervix (to protect the colon behind) and cut across the cervix at the level of the internal Os transversely.
- Send the uterus and ovaries for histological examination.
- Place a volsellum on the cervix and diathermy the endocervical canal (to ablate any residual endometrial tissue that

may have been left behind and reduce mucous production from columnar cells).

- Place a 1 Vicryl running suture from one side of the cervix to the other side to close over the cervical stump, ensuring haemostasis. Check pedicles for haemostasis.
- Close the rectus sheath with 1 Vicryl, close the skin with 2/0 Prolene. **2 marks**

7 Proceeds to explain postoperative care:

- Use of thromboembolic stockings and the need for early mobilisation; a catheter and drain will be in place for 24 hours; haemoglobin levels will be checked on day 2; skin sutures are generally removed after 5 days.
- After discharge, she will attend a follow-up visit at the outpatient clinic in approximately 6 weeks.
- Explains she will need to have regular smears until she's 65 years of age. **2 marks**

Station 13

Candidate instructions

You are asked to explain, quickly and succinctly, the meaning of the following laboratory test results and how you would manage such patients:

- Chorionic villous sampling direct preparation results: karyotype, trisomy 18
- Booking haemoglobin electrophoresis: HbSS
- Booking hepatitis B serology: surface antigen positive

Examiner's mark sheet

Chorionic villous sampling direct preparation results: karyotype, trisomy 18

1 The candidate explains these are preliminary results and that full culture results are likely to be the same in over 99% of cases; however, full culture results may differ from this preliminary result. **3 marks**

2 Explains that trisomy 18 is the second most common autosomal trisomy after trisomy 21 and is associated with a worse prognosis. Of children born with trisomy 18, 50% die within 2 months and 90% die within the first year of life. They usually suffer from severe learning disabilities and severe congenital malformations such as major heart defects – including ventricular septal defect and coarctation of the aorta – and gastrointestinal anomalies (exomphalos) that may be life-threatening. **4 marks**

3 Explains the option of a termination or of continuing with the pregnancy, but is non-directive in counselling. Explains the methods of termination if the patient wishes to know (suction termination versus medical management). **3 marks**

Booking haemoglobin electrophoresis: HbSS

1 Explains this is compatible with sickle-cell disease as opposed to trait; as such, it is more serious and has a worse prognosis. **2 marks**

2 Explains that the partner's status will need to be tested to determine the probable haemoglobin genotype of the baby. Explains that prenatal diagnosis with CVS or amniocentesis can be performed if the patient so wishes. **2 marks**

3 Explains the need to monitor this pregnancy very closely because of the increased risk of anaemia, sickle crises, IUGR, pre-eclampsia and intrauterine death. **2 marks**

4 Explains that during pregnancy the candidate would: ensure the patient is always well hydrated; reduce the risk of infections; limit the degree of anaemia; monitor her continuously during

labour; provide good analgesia – all aimed at reducing the risk of sickle crisis. Explains the use of oxygen therapy, opiate analgesics, antibiotics and intravenous hydration in the event of a crisis. **4 marks**

Booking Hepatitis B serology: surface antigen positive

1 Explain this is consistent with a hepatitis B infection at some time, although further information is required on the patient's hepatitis B eAg (if positive indicates higher infectivity) and hepatitis B e antibody (if positive indicates less infectivity) status.
3 marks

2 Explains the need to know the patient's recent liver function test results and possibly arrange for a liver ultrasound scan. **2 marks**

3 Explains that there is a small risk of vertical transmission to the baby. The candidate would allow vaginal delivery, but would avoid invasive monitoring such as fetal scalp electrodes and fetal blood sampling. Hepatitis B and C infections are not contraindications against breast-feeding. **2 marks**

4 Advises immunising the baby with hepatitis B vaccine at birth.
3 marks

Station 14

Candidate instructions

You are asked to explain, quickly and succinctly, the meaning of the following laboratory test results and how you would manage such patients:

- A 29-year old woman on day 4 of her menstrual cycle has the following blood results: free androgen index 7.9 IU/ml, LH 12.5 mU/ml, FSH 4.8 mU/ml.

- A gynaecological ultrasound report showing a right-sided partly solid, partly cystic ovarian cyst in a 47-year-old woman.

- A cervical smear result: apoptotic and ghost cells consistent with microinvasive disease.

Examiner's mark sheet

A 29-year-old woman on day 4 of her menstrual cycle has the following blood results: free androgen index 7.9 IU/ml, LH 12.5 mU/ml, FSH 4.8 mU/ml.

1 Candidate explains that the biochemical results support a diagnosis of polycystic ovarian syndrome, although this requires confirmation on ultrasound scan and existence of relevant symptoms, including oligomenorrhoea, hirsutism, subfertility, acne and obesity. **2 marks**

2 Explains that this affects around 15–20% of the female population, and, while it may cause no significant symptoms, it may be associated with a risk of diabetes mellitus in later life and a small increased risk of endometrial cancer. The candidate says s(he) would normally give her a patient-information leaflet. **4 marks**

3 Explains that treatment may include: diet; exercise; possibly metformin, oral contraceptive pill, androgen antagonists or laparoscopic ovarian drilling. **4 marks**

A gynaecological ultrasound report showing a right-sided partly solid, partly cystic ovarian cyst in a 47-year-old woman.

1 Explains that the presence of solid and cystic components are suggestive of ovarian malignancy or benign cystic teratoma. The latter is more common in younger women. It might also be an endometrioma. **1 mark**

2 The candidate says they would explore her history. In particular, how long ago this finding was made, if she has any associated pain, whether she is still menstruating (if so, it could represent haemorrhagic corpus luteal cyst, which is less significant than if she was postmenopausal), any family history of ovarian cancer or a personal history of endometriosis. **1 mark**

3 Says they would like to request tests for tumour markers, including CA125, inhibin, α-fetoprotein and estradiol to help

differentiate the type of ovarian tumour and the likelihood of malignant disease. Notes that the specificity of such markers is poor. **2 marks**

4 Explains that the ultrasound appearance is important in directing management. Says ultrasound pictures would be requested as this would enable a speculative diagnosis of the type of cyst to be made (for example, the spider-web appearance of a corpus luteal cyst, the ground-glass appearance of an endometrioma, the speckled graduated echodensities in dermoids or the papillary projections in carcinomas). **2 marks**

5 Explains that colour Doppler scanning may be of value in differentiating between benign and malignant lesions, although this is debatable. Should the cyst have a suspicion of malignancy, the candidate would discuss the findings with a local gynaecological oncologist regarding surgical management. **2 marks**

6 Explains that, depending on the patient's wishes and analysis of ultrasound films and CA125 results, surgical management could involve: ovarian cystectomy; unilateral oophorectomy with possible biopsy of the other ovary; or total abdominal hysterectomy, bisalpingo-oophorectomy and omentectomy. **1 mark**

7 The candidate explains they would have a low threshold for removing the affected ovary, with the patient's consent, and obtaining histological confirmation if there was any doubt about malignancy. At 47 years of age the biological life of the ovary is realistically 4–5 years or less. **1 mark**

Cervical smear result: apoptotic and ghost cells present that are consistent with microinvasive disease.

1 Explains the patient would be referred for urgent colposcopy (within 2 weeks) and assessment for signs of microinvasion – pollarded vessels, corkscrew vessels, large volume acetowhite, peeled rolled edges of acetowhite – and also for a repeat smear. Says that it may be wise to perform a Pipelle sample and endocervical curettage to exclude a coexisting adenocarcinoma of the cervix or uterus as glandular neoplasia is commonly present on the smear in such cases. **3 marks**

2 Explains that if microinvasion is suspected colposcopically, punch biopsies will not be sufficient and excision biopsy (wedge, LLETZ or a cone biopsy) would be preferred, otherwise microinvasion may be missed. **3 marks**

3 States that further management would depend on the excisional biopsy results:

- If < 7 mm wide and < 3 mm invasion from the basement membrane, then, providing resection margins are clear, a repeat smear and colposcopy in 6 months and 12 months time would be acceptable.

- If < 7 mm wide and 3–5 mm invasion, there is a 3% chance of nodal disease and so a radical trachelectomy (if she still wants children) or extended hysterectomy with lymph node sampling would be appropriate. **4 marks**

Station 15

Candidate instructions

You are the duty specialist registrar on call when a 36-week pregnant woman who is having convulsions is rushed in by ambulance. Explain your management.

Examiner's mark sheet

1 Candidate would resuscitate the patient: ensuring adequate airway/clearing it if necessary, giving oxygen by face mask (if she isn't vomiting), placing the patient in the recovery position in a safe surrounding where she is unlikely to injure herself, checking maternal pulse, blood pressure and oxygen saturation. The candidate would call for help (including the anaesthetist and consultant obstetrician on call for the labour ward). **2 marks**

2 Asks for relevant medical history (pre-eclampsia or a history of epilepsy), and examine the patient for signs of urinary incontinence or having bitten her tongue. **1 mark**

3 The candidate would establish an intravenous access and give magnesium sulphate 4 g in 10 ml normal saline slowly over 5 minutes, and set up a maintenance infusion (lgm/hr) of magnesium sulphate. Would consider giving intravenous antihypertensive (hydralazine or labetolol) if appropriate. **2 marks**

4 Would take blood samples for urgent full blood count, urea and electrolytes, urate, liver function tests, clotting profile and 'group and serum save'. **1 mark**

5 If the patient is still fitting after 15 minutes, the candidate would give a further bolus of magnesium sulphate 4 g in 10 ml of normal saline over 5 minutes and seek consultant assistance. **1 mark**

6 If patient is still fitting, the candidate would give intravenous Diazemuls 5 mg every 5 minutes for 15 minutes. **1 mark**

7 In the unlikely event of continued fitting, says they would consider giving intravenous thiopental. **1 mark**

8 Explains that only after the woman's observations and conditions have been stabilised would they deliver the baby. Explains that labour can be induced and vaginal delivery will be achieved in a significant proportion of cases at this gestation. **1 mark**

Station 16

Candidate instructions

Mrs Double is 21 weeks into her first pregnancy with twins. She has had no complications in this pregnancy, but would like to discuss the delivery with you. Explain how, when and why you would carry out the delivery of her twins and ask any appropriate questions that might influence your decision. The examiner may ask additional questions.

Examiner's mark sheet

1 Candidate asks whether it is a mono- or dichorionic (DC) twin pregnancy. **1 mark**

2 Candidate confirms there are no other medical, surgical or obstetric problems. **1 mark**

3 Explains that if they are monochorionic twins then the mother may need an elective lower segment Caesarean section at approximately 36 weeks to avoid the risk of acute twin–twin transfusion syndrome. Candidate is aware that the evidence base for this recommendation is weak and that the optimal gestational age for delivery is still debatable. **1 mark**

4 Explains the options of vaginal delivery or elective Caesarean section if dichorionic twins, and the pros and cons of this (higher emergency section rates for nulliparous women and risks of infection, DVT, transient tachypnoea of the newborn if elective CS). Vaginal delivery is preferable if the twin is cephalic. **1 mark**

5 Explains that if vaginal delivery is chosen for DC twins, induction of labour (IOL) would be recommended at about 38 weeks' gestation (again, the optimal gestational age) as the stillbirth rate approaches that of 43-week singletons at this point. **1 mark**

6 Explains how to deliver the second twin:
   - Give oxytocin: 2–32 U/h pre-drawn up.
   - Palpate the mother's abdomen to ensure a longitudinal lie of the second twin. An ultrasound scan may be used for this.
   - Can perform external cephalic version for a transverse and oblique lie, and allow a vaginal breech delivery of second twin if it is so presenting.
   - Aim for 30-minute inter-twin delivery interval (although this time interval is not absolute, it may be up to an hour if the cardiotocograph (CTG) is normal)
   - If the presenting part of the second twin is still high, allow descent into the pelvis provided there are no concerns for fetal wellbeing, aim to deliver in theatre/trial of instrumental vaginal delivery or an emergency CS as appropriate.

Examiner asks if the membranes of the second twin rupture and the fetal lie is transverse with its back down – how would you deliver at Caesarean section?

- Candidate says they would turn off the oxytocin infusion, try internal or external version with 0.25 mg terbutaline s.c. and attempt a breech extraction. If all fails (rare), they would perform an inverted T or J incision at CS.

- Says there is a significant risk of postpartum haemorrhage (PPH) – so would manage third stage actively and give oxytocin infusion for 4–6 hrs after delivery.   **3 marks**

7 Examiner asks if she silently dilated without contractions and delivered twin 1 at 23 weeks how would you manage her?

- The candidate would check for evidence of infection or antepartum haemorrhage, using lower genital tract swabs, clinical and biochemical signs of chorioamnionitis. If there have been no contractions for 24 hours then steroids/and rescue cerclage could be considered. Explains that this approach may delay the delivery of the second twin to improve its chance of survival, although there is no randomised evidence to recommend its routine use.   **2 marks**

Station 17

Candidate instructions

Your clinical director is concerned that there are inappropriate inductions of labour for postdate pregnancies. You have been asked to audit the number of postdate inductions of labour in your hospital. Explain in detail exactly how you would do this.

Examiner's mark sheet

1 Sets standard – RCOG guidelines recommend IOL beyond 41 weeks. **1 mark**

2 Defines audit. **1 mark**

3 Candidate understands the rationale for IOL beyond 41+ weeks and not after 43 weeks (reduce the risks of unnecessary interventions, increased workload for staff, requirement for instrumental delivery and epidural on the one hand and perinatal loss on the other). **1 mark**

4 Candidate would consult with the clinical director/audit office to determine what other questions/data to analyse. These may include the type and dose of prostaglandin used, artificial ruptures of membranes and total dose of oxytocin used. **1 mark**

5 Would determine whether audit has been performed previously and any relevant recommendations from such an audit. **1 mark**

6 Candidate would set time limits, determine specific records for analysis and consider how best to collect data. Says that the audit department may assist in obtaining notes. **1 mark**

7 Would construct an audit questionnaire to be filled out for each induction of labour (audit tool) and enter the information obtained into a computer database. **1 mark**

8 Would analyse data and compare findings to the standard. **1 mark**

9 Discusses how a change in practice may be implemented, although local policies and standards may differ from the RCOG guidelines. **1 mark**

10 The candidate would re-audit the IOL process after the change has been instituted to close the loop. **1 mark**

Station 18

Candidate instructions

Mrs Lagard is a 21-year-old French woman in her first pregnancy, and is now 20 weeks pregnant. She is referred to you with the results of a toxoplasma blood test performed 2 weeks ago at her request. She has no history of any illness and does not keep cats.

Microbiology laboratory report:

Toxoplasma IgG-positive

Toxoplasma IgM-positive.

She would like to know the significance of the test and what the possible options are for her in this pregnancy.

Examiner's mark sheet

1 The candidate gives a simple explanation of what toxoplasma is (a protozoan) and what the test means (past and recent exposure to or reactivation of toxoplasma). **1 mark**

2 Explains where the infection may have come from (cat litter or cold meats or salads). **1 mark**

3 Explains that although she has recently had toxoplasma it does not mean that her baby will either be infected or affected. **1 mark**

4 Explains the baby is less likely to be infected at earlier gestations, but if infected the consequences are usually more severe, including microcephaly, hydrocephaly, intracranial calcifications and chorioretinitis. Approximately 20% of cases are severely affected, 20% mildly affected and 60% are normal. **2 marks**

5 Explains follow-up in the fetal medicine unit to discuss further investigations, such as cordocentesis, to see if the fetus is infected. The risk of miscarriage with cordocentesis is approximately 2%. **2 marks**

6 Explains the pros and cons of medical treatment with drugs, eg spiramycin – 50% reduction of transmission with no fetal toxicity, but is less effective than other agents that are more fetotoxic. **1 mark**

7 Explains the possibility of follow-up scans to see if there are any signs of infection (microcephaly, hydrocephaly, intracranial calcifications and chorioretinitis) **1 mark**

8 Explains the worst case scenario if congenital infection occurs – there is a high risk of intrauterine death or major handicap. She could see a paediatrician to discuss the long-term prognosis. **1 mark**

Station 19

Candidate instructions

There has been an increased expenditure for prophylactic antibiotics at hysterectomy on the gynaecology ward. Describe in detail to the examiner how you would set up an audit for this.

Examiner's mark sheet

1 Candidate is aware that the RCOG standard is to give prophylactic antibiotics to all patients undergoing hysterectomy (Grade A evidence). **1 mark**

2 Defines audit. **2 marks**

3 Is aware that the exact antibiotic to be used is contentious, but this should be broad-spectrum with additional anaerobic cover. **1 mark**

4 Is aware that the duration of antibiotic therapy and the optimal route of administration is contentious. **1 mark**

5 Candidate would liaise with the clinical director, audit department, pharmacy and ward sister to devise a data sheet and see if local agreed practice or protocol meets the standard. **2 marks**

6 Would collect data sheets or put data onto a computer and analyse it over a set period. **1 mark**

7 Would analyse data to see how local practice compares with the existing standard and suggest changes or make recommendations. **1 mark**

8 Candidate would re-audit antibiotic practice after a set period of time from effecting the change to closing the loop. **1 mark**

Station 20

Candidate instructions

Describe how you would conduct the vaginal delivery of an undiagnosed breech presentation discovered during the second stage of labour.

Examiner's mark sheet

1 Candidate would ask the patient to start pushing when the cervix is fully dilated and the breech is visible at introitus. **1 mark**

2 Would offer an elective episiotomy. **1 mark**

3 If there was undue delay in descent, the candidate would consider inserting a finger in the baby's popliteal fossa to facilitate delivery of the legs. **1 mark**

4 The candidate would rotate the sacrum anteriorly with their fingers on the anterior superior iliac spines to avoid the soft abdomen. **1 mark**

5 With the scapula in view, the candidate would rotate the baby 180° clock- or counter-clockwise (Lövsett) **1 mark**

6 Would use finger to flex the cubital fossa in order to deliver the arms. **1 mark**

7 Candidate explains they would allow the breech to hang, without active traction. **1 mark**

8 The delivery would be completed by applying a mid-cavity forceps to the after-coming head. **1 mark**

9 If the head of a term baby gets stuck, the candidate would confirm that the cervix is fully dilated, apply suprapubic pressure to encourage flexion and complete the delivery with a pair of forceps. In extreme circumstances they would consider symphysiotomy, but realises, however, this is not usually advocated in the UK. **1 mark**

10 If a preterm baby's head gets stuck, an incompletely dilated cervix is usually more likely – the candidate would consider cervical incisions at the 8- and 4-o'clock positions to avoid cervical branches of uterine vessels. **1 mark**

Station 21

Candidate instructions

Mr White is angry that his wife's laparoscopic sterilisation has failed (he already has five children). You are now seeing him in the gynaecology clinic. His wife is ill with morning sickness and could not attend. It is five months since you performed the operation and she is now six weeks' pregnant. Conduct an interview with Mr White.

Instructions to role player

- Be aggressive and very upset at the failure of the sterilisation.
- Suggested questions for the role player to ask the candidate:
- Why did this happen?
- How many have you done? Why didn't a more senior doctor do the operation?
- I wasn't told this could happen, I'm going to sue you.
- I'm going to the newspapers and television.
- I'll report you to the GMC and get you struck off.
- Threaten the candidate with violence.
- Shout and raise your voice.
- Your colleagues who were assisting you were negligent as well, weren't they?
- I want compensation – how much is it worth?
- Why wasn't I given an information leaflet on this before the procedure?
- What are you going to do about it now?
- I'm not satisfied with your explanation, you don't know what you're talking about!

Examiner's mark sheet

Award marks for those candidates who display the following qualities and explain the following points:

1 Is firm, but non-aggressive, with an open posture and does not allow himself/herself to be bullied.   **1 mark**

2 Explains, using non-medical jargon, what happened and why (if possible).   **0.5 marks**

3 Says it is the patient's right if they want to take things further, and advises them that their next step would be to contact the chief executive of the trust and the complaints officer.

0.5 marks

4 Advises that if they wish to seek legal advice, that is also their right. **0.5 marks**

5 Tells the complainant they can go to the papers/TV if they wish. Realises that they (the candidate) should not talk to such representatives of the press unless directed by their defence organisation/trust press office/trust solicitors. **1 mark**

6 Explains to Mr White that he can lodge a complaint with the GMC if he wishes – he can obtain the number from the trust if he so desires. **1 mark**

7 When Mr White starts shouting, the candidate stays calm, has an open posture, does not argue, says they can empathise with his predicament – offers the correct lines of contact if he is not satisfied with the explanation (ie contacts the chief executive of the trust). **1 mark**

8 Does not implicate colleagues, even if the candidate thinks they are to blame – explains that is for an independent review panel to decide. **1 mark**

9 Does not give any cash figures as to what compensation Mr and Mrs White are entitled to, if any. Says that is for the courts to decide, if indeed liability is proven. **1 mark**

10 Explains that an information leaflet wasn't given because it is not necessarily departmental policy, although his wife may have received one. It is left to the discretion of the individual doctor obtaining the consent whether the patient needs or requires additional information. **1 mark**

11 Briefly explains the complaints procedure:
   • letter from the chief executive
   • meeting would be arranged with the consultant/departmental managers with/without the chief executive
   • independent review panel would be set up
   • settle out of court
   • settle in court
   • GMC hearing/action. **1.5 marks**

Station 22

Candidate instructions

You are given a Ventouse cup and a mannequin of a baby in a mother's pelvis, and asked the following questions:

- Explain the indications for using a Ventouse cup.
- Explain what prerequisites have to be satisfied before using a Ventouse cup.
- Explain when you would use forceps in preference to a Ventouse cup.
- Explain the possible maternal and fetal complications of the Ventouse cup.
- Explain which vacuum device you would choose and show the examiner how you would use it.
- Explain what you would do if the cup detached.
- Explain if you would convert to using forceps if the baby was not delivered after three pulls with the Ventouse cup.

Examiner's mark sheet

Explain the indications for using a Ventouse cup

1 Fetal or maternal distress, or delay during the second stage of labour.   **1 mark**

Explain what prerequisites have to be satisfied before using a Ventouse cup

1 Explains that, ideally, the cervix should be fully dilated, with no more than one-fifth of the fetal head palpable per abdomen, membranes should be ruptured, the presentation should be cephalic, the maternal bladder empty and the presenting part should be at the level of the spines or below.   **1 mark**

Explain when you would use forceps in preference to a Ventouse cup

1 Explains that the Ventouse cup and similar vacuum instruments are often considered first choice for assisted vaginal delivery over forceps because they are associated with less maternal trauma. The fetal and maternal outcomes in the long term are, however, similar.

2 Explains that if there is a large caput, poor maternal effort, inefficient suction pressure or the gestational age of the fetus is < 34 weeks then forceps should be considered.   **1 mark**

Explain the possible maternal and fetal complications of a Ventouse cup

1 Maternal – trauma to the bladder, urethra, uterus, cervix, vagina; and haemorrhage.

2 Fetal – scalp trauma/laceration, but rarely necrosis; cephalohaematoma, anaemia, jaundice, subgaleal haemorrhage, alopecia in infancy and retinal haemorrhage.   **1 mark**

Explain which vacuum device you would choose and show the examiner how you would use it.

1 Silastic/soft cup would be used for a flexed, synclitic head in an occipitoanterior position.

- Malmstrom for occipitoanterior/transverse positions.
- Bird for occiput posterior positions.
- Kiwi cup for occipitoanterior/transverse/posterior positions.

2 Seeks maternal consent.

3 Places the mother in the lithotomy position, cleans and catheterises her.

4 Re-examines to determine the position of the head and checks that is low enough to contemplate vaginal delivery:

- Explains the anterior fontanelle diamond and posterior fontanelle triangular shapes.
- They would also try to feel for an ear, to determine the baby's position especially if moulding is present.

5 Chooses a cup of an appropriate size and design, and tests it.

6 Carefully applies the cup at the flexion point (2–3 cm in front of the posterior fontanelle in line with the sagittal suture), checks that no vaginal or cervical tissue is caught up in the cup, then increases pressure up to a maximum of $0\cdot8$ kg/cm^2.

7 Explains that when a contraction is present they would employ a steady pull in line with the pelvic axis while positioning their left hand over the cup to judge the baby's descent.

8 Explains they would expect descent of the head with each pull and if not they would reconsider their decision for a vaginal delivery.

9 Candidate would expect delivery to occur or be imminent after three pulls with contractions and usually over a maximum of 15 minutes. **4 marks**

Explain what you would do if the cup detached

1 Candidate explains they would consider why it detached. Cites incorrect placement of the cup, incorrect axis of traction, poor suction pressure, large caput, head too high as reasons.

2 Says that if descent occurred with the pull they would consider reattaching the cup, but not more than twice and providing there had been progressive and adequate descent of the fetal head.

3 Explains the delivery may also be completed with a pair of forceps if descent and rotation had been achieved with the Ventouse cup. **1 mark**

Would you convert to using the forceps if the delivery is not accomplished after 3 pulls with the Ventouse?

1 Explains they would not routinely use two different instruments to deliver the baby. However, if the baby's head had descended very low in the pelvis and was in a favourable position, especially where adequate suction pressure was not achievable there was poor maternal effort or poor contractions, the delivery could be completed with forceps.

2 Explains that a Caesarean section at full dilatation with the head very low in the pelvis may cause more complications than forceps. **1 mark**

Station 23

Candidate instructions

You are asked to explain the pros and cons of hormone replacement therapy to this role-play patient. She has been referred by her GP to see you in the outpatient department.

Role player's instructions

- You are a 47-year-old married woman who has not had a period for 10 months.
- You have hot flushes and night sweats.
- You are undecided whether you want to go on HRT or not.
- You tend to go to the toilet more frequently than you used to (around 10 times per day), sometimes don't make it in time and occasionally leak urine when you cough or sneeze. You wonder whether HRT may help with your urinary symptoms.
- You have had an appendicectomy.
- You are not taking any medications.
- You smoke 10 cigarettes a day, and have the occasional alcoholic drink.
- Your mother died from breast cancer.
- Please ask the candidate the following questions:
  - Am I menopausal?
  - Will HRT improve my symptoms?
  - Will I get breast cancer?
  - Should I take HRT, and if so which route would you advise and how long should I take it for?

Examiner's mark sheet

1 Candidate introduces themselves, maintains eye contact and listens to the patient. **1 mark**

2 Takes an appropriate history:
- Asks about her menstrual history, any postcoital bleeding, date of her last smear, method of contraception and explore chance of pregnancy.
- Asks about her medical history, including risk factors for cardiovascular disease or osteoporosis.
- Asks about family history of deep-vein thrombosis (DVT), breast or endometrial cancer.
- Enquires about her social history, including smoking, alcohol and recreational drugs (how much, how often?) **2 marks**

3 Explains that the absence of periods for 1 year without pregnancy with the range of symptoms that the patient currently has would be suggestive of the menopause. Strictly speaking though, she is in the climacteric phase. **1 mark**

4 Explains that HRT may help to reduce her hot flushes, night sweats and possibly urinary urgency, although it will not reverse urinary stress incontinence. **1 mark**

5 Explains that the risk of breast cancer is increased by taking HRT (from 45/1000 to 90/1000) and more in women with first-degree relatives affected by breast cancer. **1 mark**

6 Explains that the decision to take HRT is entirely that of the patient, although there are well-documented advantages including:
- Reduction in the risks of osteoporosis, colon cancer and Alzheimer's disease, aches and pains; improvement of moods, skin, hair and teeth.
- Risky associated with HRT use, which include:
  - an increase in the risk of deep vein thrombosis from 10/100 000 to 30/100 000 and that of breast cancer after 8 years of use.
  - An increased risk of stroke and cardiovascular disease with certain continuous combined oral preparations. The

candidate explains they cannot be certain if such risks are present with estrogen-only therapy.　　　**3 marks**

7　Explains that HRT can be administered orally, or via a skin patch, gel, nasal spray or a subcutaneous implant. Explains the pros/cons of the various routes: first-pass liver metabolism with tablets, tachyphylaxis with implants, dose-metered devices with spray and gels. Also explains the vaginal route of administration with pessaries/creams and estrogen-containing rings.　**2 marks**

8　Explains that the optimal duration for HRT is currently debatable, although a duration of 4–8 years has been suggested for bone protection.　　　**1 mark**

Station 24

Candidate instructions

You are the specialist registrar on-call and have been asked to see Mrs Smith, who is 40 weeks' pregnant and has not felt the baby move today. The sonographer, who cannot see a fetal heart motion on scan has diagnosed an intrauterine death, and called you to explain the scan findings to Mrs Smith. How would you counsel Mrs Smith, who is played by an actress?

Role player's instructions

- You are a 28-year-old woman in your first pregnancy.
- This pregnancy was uneventful until today when you haven't felt your baby move.
- You are absolutely distraught at what has happened. You cry repeatedly and ask why this has happened.
- You ask what is the next step? Do I need a Caesarean section now?
- Ask why has the baby died?
- Ask if this will happen to me again?

Examiner's mark sheet

1 Candidate introduces himself/herself, makes good eye contact, comforts the patient appropriately, asks if her husband is coming and if there is anyone else she would like to be contacted, and is able to break the news to the patient and express sympathy. **2 marks**

2 Explains there is no obvious cause for what has happened. Tells the patient they would like to take some blood for tests. Says it would be helpful to conduct a postmortem examination to find out what caused her baby to die, but emphasises that the parents' permission would be needed before doing so. **2 marks**

3 Explains what now needs to be done:
- Discusses the induction process and explains that a Caesarean section is generally not recommended as it is more risky to the mother's health.
- Explains that she would be given pessaries (prostaglandins), and she would give birth in a private room on the labour ward. **2 marks**

4 Offers the services of a religious representative of her faith, if appropriate, and the phone number of a counsellor and support groups. **1 mark**

5 Explains that it is routine practice to obtain a picture of the baby and footprints, which will be kept in the notes, and that she and her husband can view this at a later date if they so wish. **1 mark**

6 Discusses her next pregnancy, as it is unlikely there will be any problems in any future pregnancies. Says she will be given a six-week, follow-up appointment with the consultant to review all the results of the investigations. **2 marks**

Answers to Paper 1 MCQs

1 F   2 T   3 F   4 F   5 T

The incidence of mild, moderate and severe dyskaryosis is 5, 1 and 0.5%, respectively. The cervical screening programme targets women between 20 and 64 years of age.

6 T   7 T   8 T   9 T   10 F

The aetiology of anal sphincter injury is multifactorial and vaginal delivery is a significant aetiological factor. Episiotomy, particularly midline episiotomy, is a significant risk factor, as well as fetal macrosomia, the use of forceps over a Ventouse, occipitoposterior position, and a prolonged second stage. Elective Caesarean section has been shown to reduce the risk of anal sphincter injury, but there is evidence that occult anal sphincter injury can occur after Caesarean section during the second stage.

11 T   12 F   13 T   14 F

Faecal incontinence is commoner in women than in men, and the incidence increases with age. Anal sphincter injury after vaginal delivery is the most significant aetiological factor. Pudendal neuropathy recovers in the majority of women after vaginal delivery and is not related to symptoms.

15 F   16 F   17 T   18 F

There is no evidence that faecal incontinence after delivery is reduced by elective episiotomy. Risk factors for the development of symptoms after a history of a previous third-degree tear include vaginal delivery in a symptomatic women, a presence of a sphincter defect of greater than one quadrant, and an increment of less than 20 mmHg on anal squeeze pressures.

19 F   20 F   21 F   22 F

Conservative therapy should always be considered in the first-line management of stress incontinence. However, the success of pelvic floor exercises is variable – reported at between 27 and 90% – and dependent on patient compliance and motivation. Most studies have not reported long-term success rates. α-Agonists have moderate effects but are not routinely used, and their use is limited by side-effects. Estrogen therapy has not been shown to be of use in women with stress incontinence. Electrical stimulation acts by stimulation of the pudendal nerve leading to contraction of the pelvic floor.

23 F   24 T   25 F   26 T   27 F

An anterior repair should not be considered for the treatment of stress incontinence. The tension-free vaginal tape procedure has a similar 5-year success rate as Burch colposuspension. Burch colposuspension, but not the Marshall–Marchetti–Krantz procedure, will correct a coexistent cystocele. Needle suspension procedures have a low long-term success rate of approximately 18%.

28 F   29 F   30 T   31 F   32 T

Premature ovarian failure occurs in 1% of women under 40 years of age. The majority of cases are idiopathic, but it is also related to chromosomal disorders (eg Turner's syndrome, gonadal dysgenesis), metabolic defects (galactosaemia, 17α-hydroxylase deficiency), immunological disorders (DiGeorge syndrome), and autoimmune disorders (pelvic tuberculosis and mumps oophoritis). Pelvic surgery and chemotherapy or radiotherapy will also lead to premature ovarian failure. Primary amenorrhoea is seen in 25% of cases. It occurs in 15% of patients with secondary amenorrhoea.

32 T   33 F   34 F   35 F   36 F

One-third of cases of azoospermia are due to non-obstructive causes, and these cases should have karyotyping performed. The other cases are due to obstruction, and in these cases a testicular biopsy usually shows normal spermatogenesis. Azoospermia is reported in 15% of infertile men.

37 F   38 T   39 F   40 F

The frequency of malignant tumours is 13% in premenopausal women and 45% in postmenopausal women. Mature cystic teratomas are the commonest tumours leading to torsion, occurring in 3.5–10% of cases. Some 2% of ovarian torsions involve ovarian malignancy.

41 T   42 T   43 T   44 T

Rupture occurs most commonly on day 20–26 of the ovarian cycle. Haemorrhage into a cyst is more common on the right than the left side, possibly due to cushioning of the left ovary by the rectosigmoid colon or the increased intraluminal pressure on the right side from the differential ovarian vein anatomy. Excessive bleeding may cause haemolytic jaundice.

45 F   46 T   47 T   48 T   49 F

The risk of ovarian hyperstimulation syndrome is related to young age, low body weight, polycystic ovaries, high dose of gonadotrophins, large number of retrieved oocytes, high estradiol level on the day of HCG administration, use of luteal support and ensuing pregnancy.

50 T   51 T   52 F   53 F

The ectopic pregnancy rate varies between 2 and 11% and a heterotopic pregnancy is estimated to occur in 1% of IVF pregnancies.

54 F   55 T   56 T   57 F

The ovulation rate in a normally estrogenised woman is reported at between 60 and 85%. The use of clomifene citrate is associated with a 50% increase in endogenous FSH and LH.

58 F   59 T   60 F   61 F

GnRH analogues are synthesised by substitution of amino acids at positions 6 and 10 of the decapeptide GnRH. After an initial increase in gonadotrophin and estrogen levels, most women will be hypoestrogenic after 2–3 weeks of starting treatment.

62 T   63 F   64 F   65 T

In the situation of 21-hydroxylase deficiency the precursor 17-hydroxyprogesterone accumulates and diverts precursors to androgen synthesis, leading to increased levels of urinary pregnanetriol, ketosteroids and serum testosterone. Aldosterone synthesis is defective.

66 F   67 T   68 T   69 F

Endocrine changes associated with the menopause include a decrease in estrone, estradiol, and androstenedione. Gonadotrophin, cholesterol and calcium levels increase, but there is no change in plasma testosterone.

70 T   71 F   72 T   73 F   74 T

Turner's syndrome is the commonest sex-chromosome abnormality. Its phenotype is related to the loss of sex-chromosome material – short stature, coarctation of the aorta, broad chest, widely spaced nipples and renal anomalies such as horseshoe kidney. Due to ovarian dysgenesis the gonadotrophin levels are raised and estrogen levels are decreased. There does not seem to be a relation with increased maternal age.

75 F   76 T   77 T   78 T   79 F

Secondary causes of hyperprolactinaemia include hypothyroidism and drugs that interfere with dopamine synthesis, release or re-uptake. It is also seen in association with renal failure and acromegaly. Around 20% of patients will have non-functioning pituitary adenomas, which increase prolactin levels by stalk compression rather than an increase in secretion.

80 F   81 F   82 T   83 F   84 T

Well-controlled diabetes mellitus and treated thyroid disease are not associated with recurrent miscarriage. Balanced or reciprocal translocations are the most frequently detected parental chromosomal abnormality. Robertsonian translocations are less frequent, occurring in 1% of couples with recurrent miscarriage.

85 T   86 T   87 T   88 F   89 T

Precocious puberty is defined as the onset of puberty before the age of 8 years in girls and before the age of 9 years in boys. Causes of precocious puberty: idiopathic (family history and overweight/obese); intracranial lesions, gonadotrophin-secreting tumours, congenital brain defects (neurofibromatosis, third ventricle cysts), hypothyroidism; and gonadotrophin-independent conditions, such as congenital adrenal hyperplasia, Cushing's disease, McCune–Albright syndrome, sex-steroid secreting tumours (adrenal or ovarian), chorion epithelioma and exogenous estrogen ingestion/administration.

90 F   91 F   92 F   93 T   94 T

Total serum testosterone levels are only raised in 40% of women, and levels do not correlate well with the severity of hirsutism or acne. The dehydroepiandrosterone sulphate (DHAs) level reflects adrenal androgen secretion and is normal in over 50% of cases.

95 T   96 T   97 F   98 F   99 T
The half-life is approximately 19 hours. The failure rate is dependent on age, being almost as low as that for the combined pill in those over 35 years of age. The failure rate is higher in those over 70 kg; therefore such women should be advised to take two pills per day.

100 T   101 F   102 T   103 T   104 F
Hyperthyroidism and hypogonadism are associated with osteoporosis.

105 T   106 T   107 F   108 T   109 T
Pathological hyper prolactinaemia may be caused by drugs that inhibit dopamine action or production, eg phenothiazines, butyropherones, methyldopa, cimetidine and pimozide.

110 T   111 F   112 T   113 F   114 F
Gonadotrophin levels are lower in Kallmann's syndrome, anorexia nervosa and McCune–Albright syndrome.

115 T   116 F   117 F   118 F   119 F
There is much experimental evidence for the aetiological role of certain high-risk human papillomaviruses – HPV 16, 18, 31, 33, 35, 45, 51, 52, 58 and 59. The HPV viruses are non-enveloped DNA viruses. Regions E6 and E7 code for oncoproteins that interfere with cell-cycle regulation.

120 F   121 T   122 T   123 T   124 F
Risk factors include early age at first intercourse, multiparity, multiple sexual partners, other genital tract neoplasia, previous CIN, combined oral contraceptive (COC) and certain dietary factors.

125 F   126 F   127 T
Cervical intraepithelial neoplasia may affect the gland crypts and the epithelium. The mean depth of crypt involvement is 1.25 mm.

128 T   129 F   130 F   131 T   132 T
Only 50% of patients show a glandular abnormality on cytology. In two-thirds of patients there is an invasive squamous lesion or CIN.

133 F   134 F   135 T
40% of women are under 40 years of age. Between 20 and 45% of patients are asymptomatic.

136 T   137 F   138 T   139 T
In patients with atypical hyperplasia, a coexistent carcinoma is found in 25–50% of cases. Cystic hyperplasia is a common fnding with risk of progression to endometrial carcinoma of 0.4–1.1%.

140 T   141 F   142 T   143 F   144 F
The risk of progression of vulvar intraepithelial neoplasia (VIN) is 5–10%. Paget's disease is associated with concomitant genital tract malignancy in 20% of cases. The risk of malignant transformation of lichen sclerosus is 3–5%.

145 T   146 T   147 F   148 F   149 F
Stage I lateralised lesions may be managed with a wide local excision. In superficial lesions the groin nodes do not need to be removed, as they are rarely involved. Elderly women have a higher incidence of nodal disease.

150 T   151 T   152 T   153 T
Malformations associated with DES exposure include a classic T-shaped uterus with widening of the isthmic and interstitial portions of the fallopian tube and narrowing of the lower third of the uterus as well as non-specific uterine abnormalities with changes in the cavity.

154 F   155 F   156 T   157 F   158 T
Krukenberg tumours occur as secondaries from primary tumours in the gastrointestinal tract, eg stomach, colon, gallbladder or bile duct. They often secrete estrogen but not progesterone or gastrin.

159 T   160 F   161 T   162 T
Knowledge of toxicity of commonly used chemotherapy is essential. Cisplatin can cause ototoxicity, nephrotoxicity and peripheral neuropathy. Neurotoxicity is a common side effect with vincristine. Doxorubicin can cause cardiomyopathy leading to heart failure. This risk is close related.

163 T   164 F   165 F   166 T   167 T

Germ cell tumours include dysgerminomas, endodermal sinus tumours (yolk sac), embryonal cell tumours, polyembryoma choriocarcinomas, teratomas and mixed tumours. A Brenner tumour and endometrial tumour are of epithelial origin.

168 T   169 T   170 F   171 T

Serous cystadenocarcinoma is the commonest ovarian tumour. Psammoma bodies are noted in 30% of cases. Bilateral involvement is seen in 30–50% of cases.

172 F   173 T   174 T   175 F   176 T

5α-Reductase deficiency occurs as a result of a mutation in the short arm of chromosome 2. Virilisation occurs at puberty. Testosterone and anti-Mullerian hormone production from the testes are normal. Affected individuals have ambiguous genitalia and are born with predominantly female or ambiguous genitalia (often clitorophallus, bifid scrotum and vagina).

177 F   178 T   179 F   180 F

Old age, obesity, abdominal distension, chest infection, malignancy and jaundice increase the risk of wound dehiscence. The mass closure technique, but not tension sutures, reduces risk. A non-absorbable suture should be used as catgut loses its tensile strength over 10 days and polyglycolic acid loses most of its strength within 21 days.

181 T   182 F   183 F   184 F   185 T

The ureter is made up of three layers and lined with transitional epithelium. It is retroperitoneal in the abdomen, passes along the anteromedial aspect of the psoas major and is crossed by ovarian vessels. It enters the pelvis anterior to the sacroiliac joints and crosses the bifurcation of the common iliac artery, passes along the posterolateral aspect of the pelvis running in front of and below the internal iliac artery. It then travels in the base of the broad ligament and is crossed superiorly and medially by the uterine artery, entering the bladder at the trigone.

186 F   187 F   188 F   189 F   190 T

The bladder has a rich parasympathetic supply and this is derived from cell bodies in the grey columns of S2–4 There is little sympathetic innervation of the bladder. Parasympathetic action is mediated via acetylcholine acting on muscarinic receptors. Sympathetic nerves originate from T10–L2 and mediate their action via α- and β-receptors.

191 F   192 T   193 F   194 T   195 T
Non-closure of the peritoneum at Caesarean section is recommended as it is associated with lower postoperative febrile morbidity and less use of postoperative analgesia. Peritoneal closure increases the risk of bladder adhesions following Caesarean section. Peritoneal closure after vaginal hysterectomy is not recommended as there is no evidence from trials to date of any benefit.

196 T   197 F   198 F   199 T
The risk of malignancy in these cysts is less than 1%. Some 50% will resolve within 3 months. It may be reasonable to manage these cysts conservatively depending on the patient's symptoms.

200 T   201 F   202 F   203 T   204 F
Some 85% of viable intrauterine pregnancies show a 66% rise in α-HCG every 48 hours in the first 40 days of gestation, but only 13% of all ectopic pregnancies show this rise. A β-HCG rise of less than 50% in 48 hours is strongly associated with a non-viable pregnancy irrespective of the site of gestation. The value of serum progesterone measurement is equivocal, as there is overlap between normal and ectopic pregnancies. A level greater than 25 ng/ml is associated with a normal intrauterine pregnancy in 98% of cases.

205 F   206 T   207 F   208 F   209 F
The peak incidence is between 30 and 45 years. It is commoner in monozygotic than dizygotic twins. Dysmenorrhoea is the commonest presenting symptom affecting 60–80% and dyspareunia is reported in 25–40%.

210 T   211 T   212 T   213 T   214 T
Danazol has side-effects related to its androgenic and anabolic properties. These include weight gain, acne, oily skin, hot flushes, depression and mood changes. Skin rashes, hirsutism and deepening of the voice, leucopenia and thrombocytopenia and cholestatic jaundice are also seen, albeit less commonly.

215 T   216 F   217 T   218 F   219 T
Gestrinone has high affinity for progesterone receptors and also binds to androgen receptors, but not to estrogen receptors. It abolishes the mid-cycle gonadotrophin surge but has no significant effect on basal levels. Some 85–90% of patients are amenorrhoeic within 2 months.

220 F   221 T   222 T   223 F   224 F
The main aetiological factors for endometrial cancer are obesity, unopposed estrogen and hormone replacement. Nulliparity increases the risk two- to threefold, and late age at menopause also increases the risk. Smoking and the combined pill decrease the risk.

225 F   226 T   227 T   228 T   229 T
Patients with one or more previous pregnancies are more at risk.

230 F   231 T   232 T   233 F   234 T
A copper intrauterine device (IUD) is the most effective emergency contraception and is not contraindicated in nulliparity. It can be fitted up to 5 days after the day of earliest predicted ovulation.

235 F   236 F   237 F   238 F
The overall pregnancy rate after progesterone-only emergency contraception is 11%. It is not contraindicated in deep-vein thrombosis, unlike the Yuzpe method. Established pregnancy is a contraindication and it can be used more than once in a cycle.

239 T   240 F   241 T   242 F   243 T
Sexual intercourse and the use of spermicides with diaphragms are strongly associated with urinary tract infections. In children up to one year of age as many as 11% of girls and 12% of boys will suffer a symptomatic urinary tract infection. It is more common in non-secretors of histoblood group antigens than secretors.

244 F   245 F   246 F   247 T   248 F
The normal parameters are a residual urine volume of less than 50 ml, a first desire to void between 150 and 200 ml, and a capacity of over 400 ml. There should be no/minimal detrusor-pressure rise during filling and if the detrusor pressure rises over 15 cmH_2O this is diagnostic of low compliance. A detrusor-pressure rise on voiding of less than 50 cmH_2O with a peak flow rate greater than 15 ml/s for a voided volume of 150 ml is normal.

249 F   250 T   251 F   252 T   253 T
Although cystoscopy is not a useful diagnostic tool, it may be used to exclude other causes of symptoms. An increase in bladder wall thickness (> 5 mm) is reported in women with detrusor overactivity. The majority of cases in woman are idiopathic, but obstruction due to prostatic hypertrophy is a significant aetiological factor.

254 T   255 T   256 T   257 T
Risk factors for ectopic pregnancy include previous tubal pregnancy and surgery, previous DID, current IUCD users, induced abortion, assisted conception, salpingitis isthmica nodosa, smoking, diethylstilboestrol exposure, luteal phase defects and ovulatory dysfunction.

258 T   259 T   260 F   261 T
In congenital adrenal hyperplasia the female fetus is exposed to low levels of androgen, and so partial masculinisation occurs. Complete development of male external genitalia will occur if the androgen levels are high enough.

262 T   263 T   264 F   265 T   266 F
Complete moles usually contain only paternal DNA and are therefore androgenetic. The majority of complete moles are homozygous 46XX, from the duplication of a single sperm in an ovum lacking maternal genes. Some 25% of complete moles are heterozygous, 46XY or 46XX. Partial moles are usually triploid, and an embryo may be present or inferred from the presence of fetal red cells in the villous vasculature. Partial moles can transform into choriocarcinomas.

267 T   268 F   269 F   270 F   271 T
The transverse colon is most likely to be injured during laparoscopy. In cases of bladder perforation the bladder should be repaired in two layers using polyglycolic or polyglactin sutures. Non-absorbable sutures should not be used as they increase the risk of stone formation.

272 F   273 F   274 T   275 T
Insertion of the Verrey's needle into the bladder does not require further treatment or catheterisation provided it is recognised and

the patient is voiding well. After stopping the combined pill, 98% of women will ovulate by their third cycle. Only 1% of women will be amenorrhoeic 6 months after stopping the combined pill.

276 T   277 T   278 F   279 F   280 T
Staging of cervical cancer includes cystoscopy, proctoscopy, cervical/tumour biopsy and intravenous pyelography.

281 F   282 F   283 T   284 T   285 F
Tumour size, differentiation and node involvement are important prognostic factors. Survival following surgery is closely related to tumour volume. In stage III disease the carcinoma involves the lower third of the vagina and/or extends to the pelvic side wall. Barrel-shaped tumours that expand the endocervix are associated with a higher treatment failure rate. Pelvic exenteration should be considered for central recurrences following radiotherapy.

286 F   287 T   288 F   289 F   290 F
Some 70% of women have advanced disease at the time of presentation. CA125 may be raised in both mucinous and serous tumours as well as in other non-malignant conditions. The prognosis and treatment of ovarian cancer are related to clinical stage, amount of residual tumour and the degree of tumour differentiation. Stage IV disease is defined by the presence of malignant cells in the cytological fluid of pleural fluid not just on the presence of a pleural effusion.

291 F   292 F   293 T   294 F   295 T
Bacterial vaginosis is commoner in Black than White women. The prevalence is 12–15% in UK populations. It is commoner in sexually active woman but can also be seen in virgins and lesbians. The pH is usually higher than 4.5.

296 T   297 F   298 F   299 F   300 T
Neisseria gonorrhoea is a Gram-negative diplococcus. The incubation period is short at 2–5 days. Reliable serological tests have not been developed.

301 F   302 T   303 F   304 T   305 T
The risk is increased in older women and if the uterine size is greater than expected for gestational age. The risk is increased in

those who have used the combined pill prior to evacuation as the hormones in the combined pill are probably growth factors for trophoblastic tumours.

306 F   307 T   308 T   309 F
They account for 2–4% of all ovarian tumours. Some 5–10% of cases arise in continuity with recognisable endometriosis.

310 T   311 F   312 T   313 F   314 T
Some 10% of epithelial tumours are borderline, and of these the most common are mucinous (30%) followed by serous. The 5-year survival rate for serous borderline tumours is 90–95%, while that for mucinous tumours is 81–91%.

315 T   316 F   317 F   318 F   319 T
Between 5 and 10% arise from a fibroid, and these have a better prognosis than those that arise in normal myometrium. Some 20% are seen in nulliparous women. There is no increased risk in Afro-Caribbean women.

Answers to Paper 2 MCQs

1 F 2 F 3 F 4 T
A positive family history is found in up to 50% of patients, and family studies suggest an autosomal-dominant mode of inheritance. The risk of stillbirth does not correlate with the level of serum transaminases, but it may be related to the maternal serum concentration of bile acids. Doppler studies are not useful in predicting fetal risk.

5 F 6 F 7 T 8 T 9 T
Pathological adherence of the placenta – as in placenta accreta, increta or percreta – is associated with previous surgical procedures to the uterus, including Caesarean section and uterine curettage.

10 F 11 F 12 F 13 F 14 T
Fetal alcohol syndrome is associated with the characteristic facies of microcephaly, growth retardation, renal and cardiac abnormalities and mental retardation.

15 F 16 T 17 F 18 T
ITP is an autoimmune disease causing purpura during pregnancy. It is confirmed by the presence of an increased number of megakaryocytes in the bone marrow. Bleeding problems are unlikely unless the platelet count falls below 50,000/mm^3.

19 F 20 T 21 T 22 T 23 T
The umbilical vein carries oxygenated blood from the placenta to the fetus. It then flows through the liver to the ductus venosus and then the inferior vena cava. Blood then passes through the foramen ovale into the left atrium before it is ejected from the left ventricle into the ascending aorta. Deoxygenated blood returns to the placenta via the umbilical artery.

24 T   25 F   26 F   27 T   28 F

A raised serum maternal α-fetoprotein level may be found in women with exophthalmos, gastroschisis and Turner's syndrome. It may also be raised after fetomaternal transfusion, eg after a threatened abortion or amniocentesis. It is reduced in Down's syndrome pregnancies.

29 T   30 F   31 F   32 F   33 T

Routine second-trimester anomaly scanning in the UK detects 25% of cases with congenital defects, 30–50% with trisomy 21. It almost never detects cerebral palsy.

34 T   35 F   36 T   37 T   38 F

Neonatal jaundice in the first 24 hours after birth is due to blood group incompatibility. Jaundice is associated with galactosaemia where there is a deficiency of galactose-1-phosphate uridyltransferase. Phenylketonuria is not associated with jaundice. Sickle-cell disease may cause jaundice in the older child but not in the neonate. Neonatal jaundice is also seen in association with hypothyroidism.

39 F   40 F   41 F   42 T   43 T

CMV is the commonest cause of congenital infection in the UK, and is commoner in lower socioeconomic groups. Infection can occur via perinatal transmission, sexual transmission and from blood products. Transplacental passage can occur in both primary and secondary infections. The highest risk of transmission is when infection occurs during the first trimester. Only 5–10% of babies infected with CMV at birth are symptomatic.

44 F   45 F   46 T   47 T   48 T

Face presentation occurs in 1:1500 births. Face presentation results in the presentation of the submentobregmatic diameter at the pelvic brim – the diameter of which is similar to occupitofrontal diameter of a deflexed vertex. The mentoanterior position is more favourable for vaginal birth. Face presentation is associated with anencephaly, pelvic malformation and prematurity.

49 F   50 F   51 T   52 F   53 F

The plasma volume increases by 50% in pregnancy and the red cell mass by 18%. Ferrous sulphate causes more gastrointestinal side-effects than ferrous gluconate. There is no evidence that routine iron supplementation improves the pregnancy outcome for women on a healthy diet, but it may do so in those in developing countries where there is a higher level of maternal anaemia. There is no effect on the risk of postpartum haemorrhage, pre-eclampsia and antepartum haemorrhage.

54 F   55 T   56 F   57 T   58 F
Congenital adrenal hyperplasia has an autosomal-recessive mode of inheritance. Marfan's syndrome and familial hypercholesterolaemia have an autosomal-dominant pattern of inheritance.

59 F   60 T   61 F   62 T
A loud, third heart sound will be detected on auscultation, not on an electrocardiogram. The PR interval is not changed.

63 F   64 T   65 F   66 F   67 T
The cerebellum is abnormal in 70% of cases. Some 95% of babies with neural tube defects have abnormalities of the head such as hydrocephalus, abnormal head shape (lemon-shaped) and abnormal cerebellar shape (banana-shaped). The maternal serum acetylcholinesterase level is normal in a closed spina bifida but raised in an open neural tube defect. Antenatal limb movement is not a good predictor of limb function postnatally.

68 T   69 F   70 T   71 F   72 F
Fetal breathing movements are increased by maternal caffeine and glucose intake. At 26 weeks' gestation the normal fetus spends 8% of its time breathing when it is active and 2% when quiet: at 34 weeks' gestation, 34% and 26%, respectively; and at 40 weeks, 28% and 16%, respectively. A biophysical profile is less accurate in predicting fetal compromise in cases of maternal diabetes than pregnancies complicated by other pathologies as the increase in amniotic fluid seen in diabetes overrides the other markers. Fetal breathing movements usually decrease 72 hours prior to the onset of labour due to fetal arterial prostaglandin E levels.

73 T   74 F   75 F   76 T
The umbilical artery waveform indices are dimensionless. They are independent of the angle of insonation. The resistance index is dependent on the maximum frequency shift during diastole (A), in diastole (B) and is calculated as A–B/A. The resistance index is 1 when there is reversed or absent flow.

77 F   78 T   79 F   80 T   81 F
Hyperthyroidism occurs in 0.2% of pregnancies and hypothyroidism in 2.5% of pregnancies. Thyroid peroxidase antibodies are associated with hyperthyroidism. There is a 50% chance of postpartum thyroid dysfunction if a woman has thyroid peroxidase antibodies in early pregnancy.

82 T   83 F   84 F   85 T   86 F
There is no indication for measurement of cervical length in a woman with a previous first trimester miscarriage or after a previous LETZ or cone biopsy.

87 T   88 T   89 F   90 F   91 F
Maternal sex steroids predominate in the fetal circulation. The fetus synthesises its own insulin and controls its own thyroid and adrenal function.

92 F   93 F   94 T   95 F   96 F
Vesicovaginal fistulas are more common than rectovaginal ones. They usually present between day 3 and 10 after the devitalised area has sloughed off. Fistulas should not be repaired immediately as some will close spontaneously. They should be managed conservatively for up to 8 weeks to allow spontaneous closure; and also to let any infection and oedema settle, which, of course, increases the chance of successful healing of any surgical procedure. The route of surgery depends on the surgical access achievable: a suprapubic route should be used when vaginal access is difficult. The success of fistula repair is related to good surgical technique and healing.

97 F   98 F   99 T   100 F   101 F
Shoulder dystocia occurs in 1 in 300 deliveries. It occurs when the bisacromial diameter is greater than the pelvic inlet. The risk of recurrence is < 5%. Since only 20% of shoulder dystocia cases occur in babies weighing over 4 kg, estimated fetal weight is therefore not a strong predictor.

102 F   103 F   104 T   105 T   106 T
In pre-eclampsia the endovascular trophoblast invasion is defective while the interstitial trophoblast invasion is normal. There is an increased sensitivity to angiotensin II. It is thought there is a decrease in fetal tolerance to paternally derived antigens. Avoidance of barrier methods of contraception and a longer period

with the same partner reduces the risk as this may increase exposure to paternal antigens in sperm.

107 F   108 T   109 T   110 F   111 F
The Korotkoff sound V corresponds best with intra-arterial pressure and is the most reproducible endpoint in pregnancy. Calcium
supplementation at a dose of 2 g/day has been shown to reduce the
risk of pre-eclampsia, but it has no effect on perinatal mortality
rates. Large randomised trials have shown little or no therapeutic
benefit of low-dose aspirin. However, a sub-analysis of the CLASP
(Collaborative low-dose aspirin) trial showed that low-dose aspirin
taken before 16 weeks' gestation reduces the incidence of early-
onset pre-eclampsia in high-risk women.

112 F   113 F   114 F   115 T   116 F
0.9% saline is the fluid of choice as 5% dextrose can result in
hyponatraemia. A metabolic alkalosis is characteristically seen. As
human chorionic gonadotrophin (HCG) is a weak thyrotrophin
agonist it may result in a rise in tetraiodothyronine (T_4) and a
lowering in thyroid-stimulating hormone (TSH) early in pregnancy. These levels normalise as pregnancy progresses and HCG
levels decrease. Unless there are clinical signs of hyperthyroidism
the patient does not require treatment.

117 T   118 T   119 F   120 T   121 F
Azathioprine, steroids, and 5-aminosalicylic acid are safe to use
during pregnancy. If the disease is well-controlled then pregnancy
does not worsen it. However, 60% of patients will continue to have
symptoms if active disease is present at the time of conception.

122 F   123 T   124 F   125 F   126 T
Local anaesthetics block conduction in Aδ-fibres at concentrations lower than needed to block C-fibres. The reverse is seen
with opioids. Epidural doses of local anaesthetic are 10 times
higher than those required for spinal anaesthesia. Dural puncture
occurs in < 1% of patients, 70% of whom will develop a severe
low-pressure headache due to CSF leakage.

127 F   128 T   129 F   130 T   131 F
Smoking is related to a decreased risk of pre-eclampsia. It also
causes a decrease in fetal breathing movements but not blood flow

to the brain. Smoking increases the risk of placental abruption and placenta praevia. The risk of miscarriage, preterm labour and intrauterine growth retardation is related to smoking in a dose-dependent fashion. It is not associated with fetal hypoglycaemia.

132 F   133 T   134 F   135 T   136 T
Type-1 diabetes complicates 1 in 300 pregnancies. Rapid normalisation of the blood glucose level in pregnancy causes a transient progression in retinopathy. The prepregnancy control, the speed of control, and extent of pre-existing retinopathy are related to the risk of progression. There is a close relationship between intrapartum glucose control and fetal hypoglycaemia.

137 F   138 T   139 T   140 F   141 F
The risk of congenital, but not chromosomal abnormalities is increased. Uterine artery blood flow is not affected by glycaemic control, nephropathy or vasculopathy. Fetal Doppler measurements are of limited value as in these pregnancies there is not the redistribution of flow seen in cases of intrauterine growth restriction.

142 F   143 F   144 F   145 T   146 F
Some 15% of cases occur during the second trimester. HELLP (haemolysis, elevated liver enzymes, low platelet count) syndrome complicates 20% of cases of severe pre-eclampsia. In 15% of cases with HELLP there is no hypertension or proteinuria. The coagulation parameters of prothrombin time, partial thromboplastin time and serum fibrinogen time are usually normal. Mode of delivery has been shown to affect transaminase levels with levels rising more after caesarean section than vaginal delivery. The recurrence rate is 19–27%.

147 F   148 F   149 F   150 F   151 F
The sampling failure rate is < 2% and the culture failure rate is as low as 0.3%. Chorioamnionitis complicates up to 1% of cases and is a cause of miscarriage. Amniocentesis is not associated with limb deformities.

153 T   153 F   154 F   155 F   156 T
A fetal heart rate of 120/minute and a respiratory rate of 30/minute each have an Apgar score of 2. Pallor scores zero. Irregular respirations score 1. Reflex activity is tested by grimace on stimulation, not the Moro reflex.

157 T   158 F   159 T   160 T   161 F

Monochorionic twins are monozygous not dizygous. There is a 10–15% risk of fetofetal transfusion, and hence an increase in the risk of fetal brain lesions and cerebral palsy.

162 F   163 F   164 T   165 T   166 F

Asymptomatic bacteriuria is seen in 3–8% of pregnant women. It is not more common in pregnancy but it is more likely to progress to symptomatic infection. If left untreated there is a 25% chance of symptomatic infection and pyelonephritis. As there is an association with preterm delivery and low birth weight it is standard practice to routinely screen women at each antenatal visit.

167 F   168 T   169 F   170 T   171 T

Some 12% of parous women are non-immune. Congenital deafness is noted even with late infection up to 20 weeks' gestation.

172 F   173 T   174 T   175 T   176 F

Continuous-wave Doppler is a blind investigation, whereas colour Doppler allows identification of the uterine artery and is therefore more accurate and reproducible. With increasing gestational age there is a reduction in resistance to blood flow within the uterine arteries. This is seen as a fall in the resistance and pulsatility indexes of the Doppler waveform, and the early diastolic notch also disappears. The high-resistance waveform persists in pregnancies where there is defective trophoblastic invasion, such as pre-eclampsia and intrauterine growth retardation.

177 F   178 T   179 T   180 F

At 6–9 weeks' gestation there is a thick septum between the two sacs of a dichorionic pregnancy, which thins but is still identifiable as a thick septum at the base of the membrane – the so-called 'lambda sign'. Dating by menstrual dates is inaccurate in 70% of cases; therefore dating by ultrasound would reduce the number of inductions performed for 'post-term' pregnancies. In spina bifida, the lemon sign is due to deformity of the frontal bone and is reliably seen up to 24 weeks' gestation. The banana sign due to abnormal cerebellar shape is seen in almost all cases from 15 weeks' gestation onwards.

181 F   182 T   183 T   184 F   185 T

Toxoplasmosis is caused by the protozoan Toxoplasma gondii and is usually asymptomatic. Some 70% of infected infants are asymptomatic but may later develop chorioretinitis, blindness, strabismus, hydro-cephaly, microcephaly, cerebral calcification, deafness and mental and psychomotor retardation. These infants should be followed up for at least two years. The risk to the fetus is related to gestational age, so if there is maternal infection there is less risk of fetal infection in the first trimester. However, if it does occur it results in more severe disease. Fetal IgM is not produced till after 19 weeks' gestation and therefore early fetal blood samples may be unreliable.

186 T   187 T   188 T   189 F   190 T
CMV infection is the commonest cause of intrauterine infection. Although it is more common following primary maternal infection, it can also occur after recurrent infection. Congenital infection can lead to growth retardation, hepatosplenomegaly, chorioretinitis, haemolytic anaemia and intracranial calcifications.

191 F   192 F   193 T   194 T   195 T
Listeria is diagnosed from cultures of blood and other sources, such as genital tract swabs and urine. It can arise from the ingestion of contaminated food such as soft cheese and paté.

196 F   197 T   198 F   199 T   200 T
Parvovirus B19 is a DNA virus. Transmission is via respiratory and nasal secretions. The rash typically appears 17–18 days after infection and after the virus is no longer present.

201 F   202 F   203 T   204 F   205 T
The majority of cases are due to trisomy from non-dysfunction caused by meiotic errors during ovum formation. Approximately 5% of cases are due to translocation where there are 46 chromosomes but one of these chromosomes is abnormal. This abnormal chromosome arises from the centric fusion of one chromosome with another acrocentric chromosome, such that the resultant child is trisomic for chromosome 21 having two independent chromosomes and the third fused to another chromosome. Increased maternal age increases the risk of non-dysfunction. If the father carries the balanced translocation then the risk of recurrence is lower than if the mother carries the translocation.

206 F   207 T   208 F   209 T
The incidence is similar in pregnancy and the non-pregnant state. The mortality rate is 17% if perforation has occurred and is higher

than in a non-pregnant woman. The diagnosis is often difficult to make and therefore treatment is often delayed. Surgery should be performed when clinically indicated even if the fetus is not viable.

210 T 211 T 212 F 213 F 214 T
Most cases of pancreatitis resolve with conservative management, and this should be the first option. Cholangiopancreatography should not be performed in pregnancy because of the high radiation risk.

215 T 216 T 217 F 218 F 219 T
Normal pregnancy is accompanied by increases in the levels of factors VII, VIII and X as well as fibrinogen.

220 F 221 T 222 T 223 T 224 T
The incidence of non-immune hydrops is 1:1000 and ratio of non-immune to immune hydrops is 9:1 The diagnosis is based on a generalised skin oedema, and collections of fluid in at least one visceral cavity. If there is only one fluid-filled serous cavity then a thick placenta should also be seen for diagnosis.

225 T 226 F 227 T 228 T
Congenital cleft lip and palate may be seen with trisomy 13 and 18 and triploidy. It is associated with the use of phenytoin and carbamazepine.

229 F 230 T 231 F 232 T 233 F
Up to 70% of patients with SLE will have a flare-up of disease during pregnancy. Anti-Ro antibodies are present in 30% of patients. Cutaneous neonatal lupus develops in 5% of babies of anti-Ro antibody-positive mothers and congenital heart block in 2%.

234 F 235 F 236 F 237 F 238 T
Symptoms of rheumatoid arthritis will improve in up to 75% of women during pregnancy. There is an increased risk of exacerbation of symptoms postpartum. Rheumatoid arthritis does not have an adverse effect on pregnancy and there is no increased risk of miscarriage.

239 T 240 F 241 T 242 T 243 T
Peripartum cardiomyopathy usually presents as heart failure late in pregnancy, the early postpartum period or up to six months' postpartum. The diagnosis is made by excluding all other causes of

heart failure. It is more common in multiparous, Black, relatively elderly and socially deprived women. In addition to anti-failure treatment, these patients require anticoagulation.

244 F 245 F 246 F 247 F
During pregnancy the plasma volume starts to increase from the first trimester by 50% of its prepregnancy level by term. Most of this rise occurs by the second trimester. The heart rate and pulse volume also increase. Diastolic murmurs are uncommon and indicate functional or anatomical cardiac abnormalities.

248 F 249 F 250 F 251 F 252 T
Engagement of the head occurs when the biparietal diameter passes the pelvic inlet. Active management of labour reduces the length of labour, but not the incidence of Caesarean section. Amniotomy does not affect the perinatal mortality rate or the operative delivery rate.

253 T 254 F 255 T 256 T 257 T
Anti-D prophylaxis should be given after a miscarriage to all RhD-negative sensitised women if > 12 weeks' gestation or < 12 weeks' gestation with heavy repeat bleeding or intrauterine instrumentation.

258 F 259 F 260 T 261 F 262 F
There is a low risk of bacterial endocarditis during delivery, but most women are also given prophylactic antibiotics to reduce this risk. These patients usually have a normal cardiac reserve. There is an increased risk of teratogenicity from warfarin use, especially between 6 and 9 weeks' gestation.

263 T 264 F 265 F 266 F 267 T
Up to 19% of fetuses with an abdominal circumference and estimated fetal weight less then the fifth centile have chromosomal defects. Some 50% of normally formed stillbirths are small for gestational age. The ratios of head circumference to abdominal circumference and femur length to abdominal circumference are poorer than abdominal circumference or estimated fetal weight alone in predicting the small for gestational age fetus or neonatal ponderal index.

268 F 269 F 270 F 271 F
The incubation period is 10–21 days. Shingles in pregnancy does not result in fetal sequelae. There is no good evidence that

varicella immunoglobulin prevents intrauterine infection. Fetal varicella syndrome may be detectable on ultrasound, but congenital varicella generally occurs after 36 weeks' gestation and has no obvious ultrasonic features.

272 F   273 F   274 T   275 F   276 T

The values of the amniotic fluid index at 28, 34 and 40 weeks are 90–220, 80–240 and 70–180 mm respectively. Amniotic fluid is increased in upper gastrointestinal obstruction due to the inability to swallow. It is increased in neuromuscular defects due to the neuromuscular loss of swallowing.

277 T   278 T   279 T   280 F   281 F

Reduced movements and hydrops can occur with anaemia from rhesus disease; however, the absence of these features does not exclude severe anaemia. The survival rate after intrauterine transfusion is 70–75% in a hydropic fetus, but 90–95% in a non-hydropic fetus.

282 T   283 F   284 T   285 T   286 T

Uterine atony is the most common cause for postpartum haemorrhage, but it can also occur due to a haemostatic defect or platelet deficiency. Fresh-frozen plasma should be given on the basis of clotting results. Most women tolerate a loss of 1500 ml before blood pressure drops. The aim of resuscitation should be to restore the circulating blood volume to a central venous pressure (CVP) of 5 cmH_2O.

287 F   288 F   289 T   290 T   291 F

Herpes gestationis is a bullous eruption in pregnancy, which clinically looks similar to herpetic lesions but is not caused by a herpesvirus. Diagnosis is made by direct immunofluorescence demonstrating C3-complement deposition at the basement membrane. Treatment is with topical corticosteroids and antihistamines. Systemic steroids are often required and should not be withheld during pregnancy.

292 T   293 T   294 F   295 F   296 F

Complication rates after Caesarean section are similar in HIV-positive and HIV-negative women. Higher viral loads lead to an increased risk of vertical transmission; however, there is no threshold value at which viral transmission will not occur. The British HIV Association recommends that combination antiretroviral therapy should be commenced if the woman herself needs treatment (ie a viral load $>$ 10–20,000 copies/ml and a CD4 count $<$ 20 $\times 10^6$) as would be recommended in a non-pregnant woman. Otherwise a twice-daily zidovudine regime should be commenced between 28 and 32 weeks' gestation, continued until delivery and also given to the infant until 6 weeks' postpartum. Breast-feeding increases the risk of transmission from 15 to 30% in UK.

297 T   298 F   299 T   300 T   301 T
In a monochorionic twin pregnancy, the death of one twin results in a 25% risk of cerebral damage and 25% risk of death in the surviving twin.

302 F   303 T   304 T   305 T   306 F
The standard deviation is the square root of the variance. The mean may be higher or lower than the mode depending on which way the data is skewed.

307 T   308 F   309 F   310 T
The following table should be constructed to calculate sensitivity, specificity and negative and positive predictive values:

	With the condition (bladder cancer)	Without the condition
Screen positive	True-positive (a)	False-positive (b)
Screen negative	False-negative (c)	True-negative (d)

The sensitivity of the test is the probability that the test is positive if the condition is present = a/(a + c) (= 50%).

Specificity is the probability that the test will be negative if the condition is absent = d/(b + d).

The negative predictive value is the probability that the condition is absent if the test is negative = d/(c + d).

The positive predictive value is the probability that the condition is present if the test is positive = a/(a + b).

Abbreviations

17 OH-P	17-hydroxyprogesterone
AC	abdominal circumference
AIS	adenocarcinoma in situ
Ag	antigen
AIDS	acquired immunodeficiency syndrome
AZT	azidothymidine (zidovudine)
bHCG	beta-HCG
BP	blood pressure
BPD	biparietal diameter
BPP	biophysical profile
BSO	bilateral salpingo-oophorectomy
C/S	culture and sensitivity (see also CS)
CA	cancer antigen
CD	cluster of differentiation or cluster determinant
CIN	cervical intraepithelial neoplasia
CLASP	Collaborative low-dose aspirin [trial]
COC	combined oral contraceptive
CPA	cyproterone acetate
CRL	crown–rump length
CS	Caesarean section (see also C/S)
CT	computerised tomography
CTG	cardiotocography
CVP	central venous pressure

CVS	chorionic villus sampling
CVT	cerebral vein thrombosis
D&C	dilatation and curettage
DAU	day assessment units
DC	dichorionic
DHA	dehydroepiandrosterone
DHEAS	dehydroepiandrosterone sulphate
DVT	deep-vein thrombosis
ECG	electrocardiogram/graphy
EEG	electroencephalogram/graphy
EFW	estimated fetal weight
EMG	electromyogram/graphy
EPAU	early pregnancy assessment units
EUA	examination under anaesthesia
FAS	fetal anomaly/abnormality scan
FBC	full blood count
FISH	fluorescence *in-situ* hybridisation
FSH	follicle-stimulating hormone
GnRH	gonadotrophin-releasing hormone
GP	general practitioner
GTT	glucose tolerance test
GU	genitourinary
GUM	genitourinary medicine
h	hour
HAART	highly active antiretroviral therapy
HbSS	haemoglobin SS
HCG	human chorionic gonadotrophin

HDU	high-dependency unit
HELLP	haemolysis, elevated liver enzymes, low platelet count [syndrome]
HFEA	Human Fertilization and Embryology Authority
HIA	haemagglutinin inhibition assay/antibody
HIV	human immunodeficiency virus
HMG	human menopausal gonadotrophin
HRT	hormone-replacement therapy
HSG	hysterosalpingography
HVS	high vaginal swab
HyCoSy	hysterosalpingo-contrast-sonography
Ig	immunoglobulin
im	intramuscular
IMB	intermenstrual bleeding
INR	International normalised ratio
IOL	induction of labour
ITU	intensive therapy/treatment unit
IUCD	intrauterine contraceptive device
IUD	intrauterine device
IUGR	intrauterine growth restriction/retardation
IUI	intrauterine insemination
iv	intravenous
IVF	*in-vitro* fertilisation
IVP	intravenous pyelogram
IVU	intravenous urography
LAVH	laparoscopic-assisted vaginal hysterectomy
LH	luteinising hormone

LLETZ	large loop excision of the transformation zone
LMWH	low molecular weight heparin
LSCS	lower segment Caesarean section
MAC	membrane attack complex/*Mycobacterium avium* complex
MRC	Medical Research Council
MRCOG	Member of the Royal College of Obstetricians and Gynaecologists
MRI	magnetic resonance imaging
MSAFP	maternal serum α-fetoprotein
MSU	mid-stream urine
NHS	National Health Service
NICE	National Institute for Clinical Excellence
NT	nuchal translucency
OA	occipitoanterior
OHSS	ovarian hyperstimulation syndrome
OT	occipitotransverse
PCOD	polycystic ovarian disease
PCOS	polycystic ovarian syndrome
PCR	polymerase chain reaction
PCT	primary care team
PE	pulmonary embolism
PET	pre-eclamptic toxaemia
PFA	plain film of the abdomen
PMS	premenstrual syndrome
PPH	postpartum haemorrhage
PPROM	preterm, prelabour rupture of membranes
RCOG	Royal College of Obstetricians and Gynaecologists

RIA	radioimmunoassay
s	second
sc	subcutaneous
SFH	stroma-free haemoglobin
SGA	small for gestational age
SHBG	sex hormone-binding globulin
SLE	systemic lupus erythematosus
T_4	tetraiodothyronine
TAH	total abdominal hysterectomy
TED	thromboembolic disease
TFT	thyroid function test
TOP	termination of pregnancy
TORCH	toxoplasmosis, other [congenital syphilis and viruses], rubella, cytomegalovirus, herpes simplex virus
TSH	thyroid-stimulating hormone
TTP	thrombotic thrombocytopenic purpura
TVS	transvaginal ultrasound
U&E	urea and electrolytes
USI	urodynamic stress incontinence
USS	ultrasound scan
VH	vaginal hysterectomy
VIN	vulvar intraepithelial neoplasia
WBC	white blood cell/count
WCC	white cell count

Index